ROCKSTARS, SHOWBIZ, THE PLAYBOY MANSION, AND BROADWAY MY BEST LIFE YET!

ROCKSTARS, SHOWBIZ, THE PLAYBOY MANSION, AND BROADWAY MY BEST LIFE YET!

Linda Hoxit

Published by Taft House Publishing.

ISBN: 9798269930176 (sc)

This book is printed on acid-free paper.

Cover design by Doug Haverty
Interior Design by Newgen
All Photos Courtesy of Linda Hoxit

For my forever role model Ann-Margret Olssen and my loving and generous husband Alan. Also, BFFs in Eternity, Sha, Bridget, Jani, Susan, Linda K., DJ, Peter, and Rrrrrroberto. The last one standing writes the book. Eternal thanks to my friend, director, and mentor, Bruce Kimmel, who has helped me every step of the way.

TABLE OF CONTENTS

INTRODUCTION

This isn't a cradle to grave memoir, rather a cradle to age 30 memoir about my life and career in the show business industry as a dancer, singer, actress, artistic swimmer, a commercial actress and model. People INTO THE DOZENS have been telling me, pushing me, requesting me to write my stories because of all of the facets and stories I have to offer. I just didn't come up with the book idea on my own.

What made this period of my life extraordinary was my personal life with two rock star boyfriends, my boyfriend Keith Hefner, Hugh Hefner's brother and living part time at the Playboy Mansion and finally originating a role on Broadway in the ill-fated stage version of *Seven Brides for Seven Brothers* as one of the seven brides.

Also, I'd like this to be an inspiration for up-and-coming girls and guys from smaller non-show business towns to assure you that if you work hard and study with good teachers you can succeed.

It can be hard and scary to leave your family and friends. And you should probably consider at least enrolling in a good college program, even a good junior college program, for a while. I must admit I never earned a full college degree in the performing arts, but I sure did need more training and mentoring and I made new friends who became my family and who I still have to this day. They were likeminded people and artistic and who I should be around anyway. So whatever reason you're reading this, I hope you enjoy and know that it is all the truth, and it's MY truth.

Linda

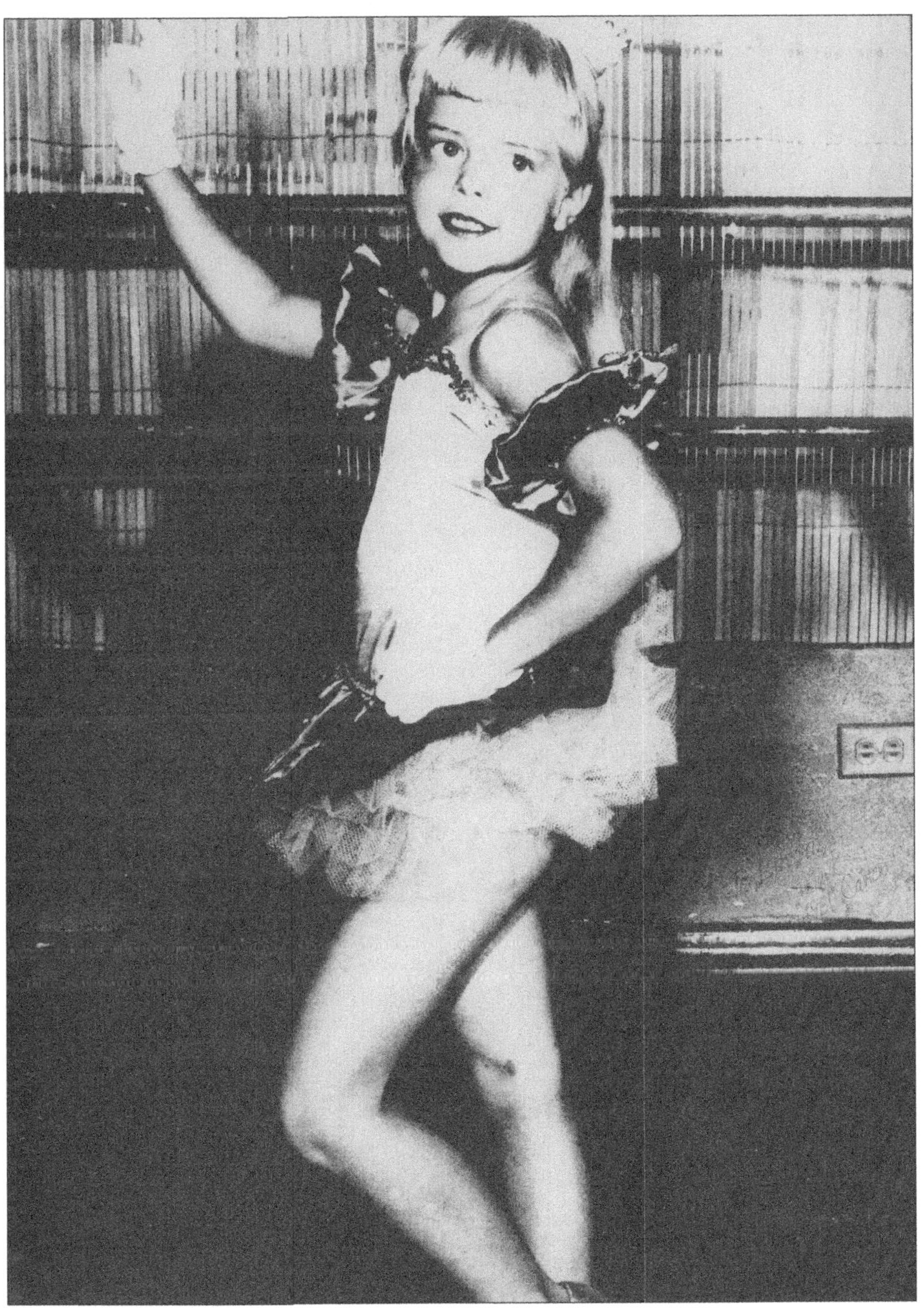

Linda 1958 “Baby Take a Bow” Shirley Temple Tap Dance

CHAPTER ONE

BORN UNDER A BAD SIGN

I was born on a blustery Friday morning, on March 13th, 1953, to parents Beverly Joyce Miller and Johnny Ray Hoxit. He was serving in the Korean War as a Navy Private first class. We were living with my mother's parents, Frieda and George E. Miller II, in the naval town of Bremerton, Washington, until my dad returned from the worthless war that that war was.

The nurses and doctors at Harrison Memorial Hospital told my mom and grandparents that I was the prettiest baby they had ever seen born there. When my dad returned from the Korean War, we moved to Bridgeton, New Jersey, where his relatives lived. Unfortunately, my dad suffered from PTSD and still had shrapnel embedded in his backside from being wounded on the front lines.

The marriage just wasn't going to work out. Eventually, mom left and moved us back to Bremerton, with my grandparents. She was also pregnant now with my sister Kathy, as we moved back.

As it turned out, it was a fortuitous living arrangement. My mom was coming down with bipolar disorder, and we would end up living with my grandparents until I graduated from high school and went to college. I still thank God for my grandparents every day for helping us. My mom continued to work and raised me and my sister with the financial and emotional help of my grandparents. Like every working single mother, she struggled with time and money to raise my sister and myself, and was receiving NO child support from Johnny Ray, as he wasn't working, and was disabled. My grandfather still worked at the National Bank of Commerce, while my grandmother was a stay-at-home grandma. They helped us tremendously. We had a comfortable large house, and a beautiful summer cabin at Hood Canal on the North Shore.

When I was four years old, it was decided by my mom and grandma that I should take dance class. In the 1950s, many moms and grandmas wanted their granddaughters to become another Shirley Temple. Fortunately for me, they chose the best dance studio in Bremerton. It was owned by Margie Speck. She had moved up from Culver City, California with her family. Margie's father worked in set construction at MGM Studios, and she had studied tap dancing with Bojangles Robinson.

I took a combination ballet, tap, and acrobat class once a week for an hour, for two years. Indeed, we learned Shirley Temple dances and songs. My grandmother would take me to ladies' luncheons at the Elks Club and Eagles Club. There I would perform solo or duo with other little girls my age and do the Shirley Temple dances and songs, dressed in full costume, with sausage curls that my grandmother had put in with rags, a style of the times, with my long blonde hair. After two years I lost interest.

I developed other interests, and my grandparents had the resources to support them. I was in Brownies and Girl Scouts, and Western style horseback riding at our cousins' riding Academy once a week between the ages of seven and nine. I got heavily involved with the Free Methodist Church and I was a Christian Crusader. I was also a voracious reader and read many books on archaeology in particular, Egyptian pyramids and culture, and was fascinated with books about World War II and the Third Reich (ha ha, at 8 years old). And of course there were Nancy Drew mysteries.

I was also given piano lessons that I could only endure for about a year. Then in grade school I studied violin. I loved my little baby violin. I loved rosining the bow. I also loved my teacher, Mr. Funk, who looked like an elf. What I didn't love was reading music. I just never clicked with it. So that only lasted from 2nd to 4th grade. Then I was put in choir, and I thrived. Like my mother, I had a strong singing voice and basically perfect pitch for my age. I could read note values and if the notes went up and down on the scale, that was easy. But to this day and after singing professionally for years, I still can't fully read music.

When I turned 10, The Margie Speck Dance Studio moved two blocks away from my home. We spent most of the summers at Hood Canal at our summer cabin, but when we came back home, I'd go down to Margie's studio and watch her advanced classes do production dances in her large parking lot. She did a great rendition of the ballet Rodeo by Aaron Copland. Her advanced dancers were quite good and very energetic.

So, from then on, I was hooked on dancing again. It was easy for me to walk to the dance studio and home again, as our neighborhood was very safe. Another reason is that it made it easy for me to become a better dancer. I didn't have to continually bug anyone for rides.

Margie was also skilled at musical theater dance, and jazz dance. She was particularly fond of *Sweet Charity* and *West Side Story*. Margie would teach herself the choreography from both movies and we would do it in class. It was good solid Bob Fosse and Jerome Robbins choreography.

The icing on the cake of taking dance from her was her command of ballet dance as well. She would go over to Seattle and study with The Ladres from Russia who had moved from Russia to Seattle and had their own dance studio. So, we received excellent technical ballet training.

When I turned 12, I went to Coontz Junior High School, then 7th and 8th grade only. Coontz's claim to fame Was that Quincy Jones went there when he lived in Bremerton for a few years before moving to Seattle. His father had come to Bremerton from Chicago to work in the naval shipyard.

Since I've been singing a lot in choirs in grade school and had a decent voice, I was put into a select choir called Troubadours. Our choir teacher was Lewayne Hoffman and what a nice man and teacher he was. We sang a lot of musical theater songs, memorably selections from *Oklahoma!* I was supposed to be an alto, but I cheated and sang the melody. I didn't quite grasp singing harmony at that time. Still, I got a great deal from the class and the teacher. It also didn't hurt that many of my girlfriends were in the class.

I was still at Margie Specks studying dance. Since we were a Naval town, we had many students come from Naval parents previously stationed at different Naval bases around the USA. They would come and go as their parents were reassigned to other bases or to Bremerton. One young woman in particular, Suzanne Williams, came in with her family when I was 13. She had superb ballet training and had won a scholarship to San Francisco Ballet School in

San Francisco, California. She changed everything for us. We all became obsessed with ballet and obsessed with winning San Francisco Ballet School scholarships. We also performed The Nutcracker ballet every December. We were the first dance studio in the Pacific Northwest to do so, so it benefited all of the serious students to take their ballet more seriously.

I started taking more ballet classes. I even came down to the studio by myself and did ballet barre and exercises. I progressed and I was chosen to be Clara in our production of *The Nutcracker* in 8th grade when I was 13. I continued to take all forms of dance that Margie offered, but my ballet and technique were really becoming strong.

I turned 14 in March of 1967, and San Francisco Ballet had their annual auditions that spring at the Cornish School of the Arts in Seattle. I did a good job. and I earned a scholarship for the summer of 1967 in San Francisco.

I also had the ability to watch what I ate and kept myself on a strict high protein diet, as ballet dancers had to be thin and lean. My grandparents and my great aunt Viola were able to scrape together enough money for me to fly down and live with a French family, the Fralis, that summer, since housing was not provided.

Boy, did I have a blast! 1967 and the Summer of Love in San Francisco. I did make it to Haight-Ashbury once or twice, but it was kind of scary. Still the whole essence of hippies and rock'n'roll was mesmerizing and addicting. I made friends in San Francisco and was popular in the dance classes. I got so much better at ballet, and at the end of the summer I was offered a Ford Foundation scholarship by Harold Christensen, director of the school. That would mean I would stay the whole year in San Francisco and have to find a place to live with a family. I was very flattered, but I just couldn't make myself do it.

Back in Bremerton, I went to live with my folks and be with my friends, plus I started high school. I was a freshman at West Bremerton High School. It was exciting. I am a big kid now! I had tried out to be a freshman cheerleader and almost made it, but it was meant to be that I never made it. About a year previous, I had decided that I wanted to make dance my career. I had thought about becoming an archaeologist, but Egypt was out of the question at the time. It had severely restricted what you could research as an archaeologist because people were abusing Egyptian artifacts, robbing Egypt of its rich history.

So back to dancing at Margie's and nose to the grindstone, as usual. I also was in the freshman choir. The choir teacher George Manske and I didn't get along. I think he was intimidated by me, actually.

He knew I was an award-winning dancer and when the school musical came along that Spring (one of my favorites, *Bye Bye Birdie*), he did not choose me. Boy, was I pissed. He only chose one freshman female because he said she was more mature. I've often thought over the years how he must have felt at not choosing me, after my hometown newspaper, the Bremerton Sun, made a big deal of all my career and dance successes.

High school was and continues to be hard on many a young person. Kids are cruel and there are still bullies, no different in 1967 and 1968. Since I was very thin and lean, I had very tiny breasts and back then the body type for young girls tended to be more T&A oriented. Some of the boys at the high school referred to me as a "pirate's treasure," a sunken chest. I needed to stay thin and learn to achieve my dance career and keep winning scholarships like I was doing, and I DID!!! Fuck 'em, huh?

CHAPTER TWO

BOYS, DRUGS, AND ROCK 'N' ROLL

Now I'm a freshman at West High School, Bremerton, navigating my way through my freshman year. One of my best friends, Teddy Tillett, had a party at her house. Her parents were party animals, too, and they let her have a live band with her sister. It was in the basement of her house, which sat up on a tall hill, and there were many steps to climb to get to the house.

When another friend and I got to the door of the basement, there were a lot of teenagers there. I finally got to a place where I could see the band. They were playing, and the lead singer was singing "My Little Red Book," by Burt Bacharach and Hal David, but more like the band Love's version. The male singer was very animated and energetic, and ... cute! He looked like Keith Partridge of

The Partridge Family, except with freckles. We continued to enjoy the band and then went home.

Back at school on Monday, I found out that Teddy was dating him. His name was Mike Gray. He was from East Bremerton, and a few years older than us. He had also been kicked out of East High School, a genuine bad boy.

I didn't think much about him, and I didn't ask Teddy much about him. But about a month later, I was at an all-city teen dance. These were dances that the city of Bremerton provided for teenagers, were relatively safe—no alcohol or drugs were allowed. Local bands like the Chimes of Freedom played at them, basically to keep all the teenagers safe and off the streets.

I was with another friend named Sue, and my eyes caught Mike standing on the side of the hall listening to the band, with another guy, not Teddy. I think his eyes caught mine looking at him and I smiled. So, Mike walked over to me and asked me for a dance, which of course I accepted. After our dance, we walked to the side, and he asked me my name. He also asked me if I was seeing any boy or had a boyfriend. Of course, I didn't, and he wanted to know if he could take me on a date the following week. I said sure, and we continued to do some dancing and some slow dancing, which I found very enjoyable. And I did find out that he and Teddy were no longer seeing each other.

Now here I must digress. I grew up in a Scandinavian household, with a grandmother that was completely Norwegian. My grandfather was completely Scottish, and my mother, of course, half and half. Scandinavians in general are very gentle and kind parents. I was never hit or spanked—yelled at yes, but never any corporal punishment. Another apparent character trait of Scandinavian parents was to not tell their kids that they were good looking. They didn't want them to grow up to be vain or narcissistic.

So, although I was a beautiful young girl, with beautiful blonde hair, NOT ONCE was I told that I was cute or pretty by my grandparents, mom, or great aunts and uncles. My dad was nowhere to be found after they divorced.

I sort of thought I was good looking, but I had no assurance of that. All I had was looking at other young girls on TV and movies and trying to compare myself with them. I felt I was pretty close, but as a result, I didn't have very good self-esteem. Combined with the teenage boys at West High School calling me a pirate's treasure, due to my flat chest, it was thrilling to have any boy ask me out, and particularly, Mike.

The following Saturday night rolls around after a week of total anticipation. Mike pulls up in a sort of "beater" car with a friend of his driving and comes up to the front door to get me. He looked very cute per usual in clothes of the day: tight pin striped pants, a dress shirt with a corduroy maroon jacket, and his long brown hair and freckled face, oh boy! My grandparents met him, but he was not asked in, and they just said hello to him, and to please have me back by eleven.

So, we went back down to the car with his friend waiting in the driveway. What most teenagers did In Bremerton on a Friday and Saturday night on their dates was to cruise town in cars. Then maybe if you were lucky, you'd stop by the local Frosty Freeze for a soft drink or a shake.

I was introduced to his friend Bruce, who was sort of a gaunt looking, thin blonde teen who seemed very sweet and sort of shy. We sat in the back seat of the compact car, close together to signify we were on a date. Bruce drove us, chauffer style, downtown to the main drag where all of the other teens were cruising with their significant others or dates. I thought it was sort of odd, sort of subservient, but Bruce didn't seem to mind. Everyone just passed each other at about three to five miles an hour and waved and sometimes honked. This went on between the hours of 7 to 10 pm.

Mike and I spoke, and he told me he still lived at home, but didn't attend East High School, as he was kicked out for fighting and being a degenerate. He had no job and no car, so his best friend Bruce would help him out on dates. He also told me how very cute he thought I was, and then he dove in to make out with me, French style, OH YEAH! His friend drove us out to a deserted parking lot where all the other teenagers went to pet and neck and we continued French kissing, but that was all for that night. After about an hour (poor Bruce) it was enough for one night, but Mike told me he wanted to go steady, and he'd come and walk me home from school on Monday.

My Norwegian grandma Frieda was up and waiting to greet me at the door. She wanted to know how things went, and I said he wanted to keep seeing me. She said she and grampa didn't like him at all because he was from the wrong side of the tracks.

I basically told her that that was not going to stop me, and she said, "Okay, but he's not going to come into the house, and he can drop you off at the front of the yard." So that's what transpired. He'd walk me home from school and then he'd stop at the driveway and walk back to his house or hang out with his friends.

This routine went on for a couple of months, walking home from school, going out on Friday or Saturday night with Bruce driving alone with no date, and us in the back seat progressively getting more and more sexual, as Mike knew what and where to touch me, and bring me to climax, although I really didn't know what that was. He wanted me to touch him as well (again, he was a bad boy), but that did not work for me, not at 14.

Homecoming and the Homecoming Dance was coming up, and I wanted to go, and Mike agreed to take me. So,

I told the parents, and I went to Seattle, to my fave teen clothing store, Jay Jacobs, and got a fancy silver mini dress with shoes to match.

On the Friday night of the dance, Mike pulls up to the driveway with Bruce, in the beater. I get all dressed up, and Mike is in his usual garb. I was like, "What's going on?" He said, "I have no money for admission to the dance, but we're going to go to Frosty Freeze and get some burgers. You don't really want to go to a stuffy old school dance anyhow, do you?" Oh, hell yes, I did, but I just said I guess not, as we drove past the high school with all the young couples all dressed up and going in with their corsages and nosegays.

He brought me home after the usual petting and foreplay with NO SEX, and that was basically our last date. It was sort of unspoken, but I'd had enough of the sexy bad boy, and about two weeks later he'd hooked up with another attractive girl that was a year older than me, which was painful to see but fine. I would not have another boyfriend for about a year or even date, but I had plenty to do to keep me busy with my dancing and schoolwork. I was a good student and enjoyed learning.

Freshman year progressed and so did my dancing. Margie did another *Nutcracker*, and I got the role of the Dewdrop Fairy, the soloist in "Waltz of the Flowers." As I said before, I auditioned for the high school musical, which was *Bye Bye Birdie*, but was not chosen because I wasn't mature enough, at 14 years old.

I auditioned again for The San Francisco Ballet for a summer scholarship and was chosen. It was now the summer of 1968. I went back and made more friends that summer, notably Amy Edelstein and John Townsend (who I dated sporadically, and who turned me on to cannabis).

Amy's sister worked at Bill Graham's Fillmore Ballroom, where all the hardcore psychedelic bands played at the time. Her name was Joanie Edelstein, and she worked concessions. The Edelstein family were also connected to the band Quicksilver Messenger Service, and Joni wanted Amy and me to come to the Fillmore the night they were playing that summer.

So, we put on our hippie finest and went!!! We walked in. It was a large space with a very high ceiling. There was a light show going on, although the band wouldn't be onstage for another forty-five minutes. "Hey Mr. Fantasy" was playing nice and loud over the loudspeakers, with the ethereal Steve Winwood singing, lead singer of the band Traffic at that time.

You could smell incense and cannabis wafting through the air. I had died and gone to hippie heaven. But about five minutes after we entered the Fillmore, Joni came to us and said, "Linda's parents called from Bremerton, and she has to go home. They don't want her being here."

Oh my God! I was put in a taxi and taken back to the boarding house where I was residing. They told the Edelstein parents that they were afraid I was around too many people dropping acid, which I hadn't done yet, and I knew my parents weren't sure what that meant! What a disappointment, but at least nobody was mad, just me.

Anyhow, I finished the summer studies with San Francisco Ballet, and once again, Harold Christiansen asked if I wanted a Ford Scholarship and I politely declined. It was time to go back to "B" town as we called it, and become a full-blown young hippie girl, with my oh so fun and wild group of friends with great senses of humor, ready to explore whatever we could.

It was sophomore year, 1968, with the hippie movement and psychedelic and cannabis drug movement in full force. Also, just the BEST music to this day: British Invasion bands like The Rolling Stones, Rod Stewart with Jeff Beck, Iron Butterfly from Los Angeles, Cream from England, the Beatles, of course, Crosby, Stills, Nash and Young, and Chicago. I saw all of them in person, either at Key Arena in Seattle, or at Eagles Auditorium.

My mother took my sister and me to see the Beatles at Key Arena four years earlier, in 1964, when I was 11 years old and my sister was 9. We were in matching white dresses with blue embroidery, and mom was in her powder blue suit, a Norwegian vison of blondes in blue. It was our very first rock concert, and what a way to begin loving live rock music, and the boys in the bands.

I will never forget when the Beatles hit the small stage, surrounded by policemen on all sides. The noise from the sold-out crowd was white noise, and the first two songs they played, "I Wanna Hold Your Hand" and "I Saw Her Standing There," were barely audible. Many female teenagers ran down to the stage and tried to jump on it, but Seattle's finest were there to grab them. One lucky girl grabbed John Lennon's leg, and we thought that it was so cool. The Beatles did a full hour set, and it was over too fast.

As we made our way out of Key Arena (it was at that time Seattle Center Coliseum) the teenage girls were crying and walking and holding one another up. Many looked ill and had visible mucus coming from their noses and mouths. My sister and I just looked at them with wide eyes and our mouths hanging open, my mom laughing as she held our hands to go back to the Bremerton Ferry Boat, our mode of travel. It was an unforgettable experience.

But back to 1968. I was fortunate to have a very nice group of girlfriends, and I don't know how we managed it, but we developed a friendship with a lovely group of older boys who liked smoking weed and going over to Seattle to the rock concerts. Terry O'Hare and Mike Pizzuto were two that came to mind. No one got involved romantically and the boys were so honorable. We were lucky to have them.

One outstanding concert was on a warm spring day in May 1968. It featured Three Dog Night opening for the British band Led Zepplin on the floating stage at Green Lake in Seattle, which is now long gone. We were soooooo stoned on weed, and both bands were just superb.

Next, there was the Jimi Hendrix concert in Seattle. He was Seattle's OWN claim to fame, who, by 1969, claimed the well-deserved title of World Class Rock Star, and a phenom to this day. I was at a party in 1969, and now a junior in high school, when an obnoxious red-haired boy from another high school asked me if I'd go see Hendrix with him. He was loud and had a sharp, pointed nose, and I didn't like him right off the bat. My two best friends were there with me, and when I told them, they said, "OH MY GOD, JUST GO, IT'S HENDRIX." So, I did and at least I did get to see Jimi.

The sharp-nosed, red-haired teenager picked me up, and, as usual, we took the ferry to Seattle, where he was even more obnoxious. We were with some of his friends, who put up with his bad jokes and sarcasm. The concert was at Key Arena like most concerts for rock music, and I can't remember who the opening act was, but there was one.

Jimi finally took the stage surrounded by cops, but the kids would NOT stop trying to jump the stage. After about four songs, the announcer/manager of the show came on and told us that if people didn't stop jumping the stage, they'd stop the show. It was just too much for the cops to deal with. Jimi made it through one more song, the teenage boys did not stop, then full lights came on, and the concert was brought to a halt, the end. The only good thing was my "date" was over. It was the worst date of my teen years. I don't remember his name, and when he asked for a kiss as he dropped me off, I told him I didn't kiss on the first date, and I never heard from him again.

My close-knit friends and I had also started dropping acid as well as smoking weed towards the last two or three months of our sophomore year in high school. My experience with that was relatively short lived, and I did have some very mind-expanding times on it, and I have no regrets doing so.

Acid was also really fun, and we laughed a lot. The thing you have to do to have a good trip is to do it with friends, to do it WITH people. I never dropped acid by myself; we'd plan group drops anywhere from three to ten people. We did it on the weekends, sometimes in the daytime, and other times at night, all night.

The most incredible time was when a group of about a dozen of us boys and girls went to the Washington coast and camped for two days. We had gorgeous weather, and we all took our dose mid-morning as it took about an hour to kick in. It was a larger tab of acid called "chocolate chip" as it sort of looked like a large, flat chocolate chip. The twelve of us walked in a straight line up and down the gorgeous ocean beach all day long, hallucinating our asses off. The colors of the sand were like spun gold. The water and tidepools were electric blue, as colors intensified on psychedelics. The hallucinogenic high lasted a good eight to ten hours before you started to come down. Then we had to go back to our little camp and cook and eat beans and hot dogs over a bonfire that we had taken from home, along with potato chips and some sort of cheap rotgut wine.

We were not into sex yet, and I was scared shitless of getting pregnant, as that was considered shameful at the time, so we did drugs instead. I compared notes years later with other teens I went to school with who admitted to already having sex by fifteen but did not do drugs.

For those of you reading this who've never taken a psychedelic drug, you don't really "see things" like objects floating around like flowers or animals in the sky. I have to laugh when over the years some TV shows and movies have portrayed that as a given, when ingesting any psychedelic drug, but I never ingested LSD 25, which may have done that.

I did "shrooms," MDMA and/or Ecstasy (my personal favorite), and last but least was mescaline. My group of friends got into mescaline and switched up from acid and the high was okay. But after coming down, I became paranoid about my friends talking behind my back, which they were not. So, I quit all psychedelics for about three years and just stuck to beer, wine, and weed when I partied. Besides, I had my career in my sights, whereas my tribe had not decided on that for themselves yet.

I kept at my dance classes but had no singing or acting yet. When the high school musical came around, I was chosen this time, as I suppose I was finally mature enough. I got a chorus part and was cast as a Hot Box Girl in *Guys and Dolls*. I loved singing and dancing in "Bushel and a Peck," and as a bitter chorine in "Take Back Your Mink." In this, I had to rip off pop beads and clothes with Velcro and throw them to the floor, uncovering a sexy, skimpy leotard and mesh tights, all while doing sexy little dance steps. Then I picked all of it off the floor at the end and headed offstage in a snit. It was too wonderful for words! I have seen *Guys and Dolls* over the years many times, and I never fail to laugh at the jokes and the hilarious writing. I was never cast in it again, though I would've loved doing it again.

That spring, something new was afoot for the greater Seattle area. Robert Joffrey and the Joffrey Ballet were coming to Pacific Lutheran University, under a newly formed program of Pacific Northwest balletomanes called Pacific Northwest Ballet Association. Robert Joffrey grew up in Seattle and trained with ballet teachers there. He was a short, muscular man with an interesting but not handsome face, and had a direct and commanding presence. He'd be holding auditions for teenagers twelve to eighteen for the Joffrey Company's summer in residence program, and for approximately forty male and female ballet dancers, who were the cream of the crop of Washington State. I auditioned and won a scholarship, so I was not going back to San Francisco Ballet as this was more prestigious and closer to home at Pacific Lutheran University in Tacoma.

The teenagers were divided into two groups. The vast majority were teenage girls and only a handful of boys. It was intimidating for me, as I was with many dancers from Seattle who were quite phenomenal, including Francesca Corkle, Ann Reinking and Theresa Padvorich, to name a few. We took daily classes, six days a week, which included character and Flamenco dance taught by a senior woman from Chicago, Edna McRae, who was Robert Joffrey's right-hand woman. I did very well in those. I struggled to keep up with some of the other dancers in the class.

We had Sundays off, and sometimes my friends would come and visit me from Bremerton, and we'd go driving around and smoke weed, but no LSD or mescaline, as it usually took a day to recover from trippin'. Drugs and drug use was quite different then. They were truly used recreationally, not daily, at least for myself and my teen tribe. The drugs of today seem to be much more addictive and dangerous, and I would never EVER consider Fentanyl or heroin, besides we never shot up drugs.

The great thing about the Joffrey Ballet was since the company was in residence for the summer, we were bused to Seattle twice to see them perform at the Seattle Opera House. My favorite ballets of the Joffrey were the bizarre "Green Door," the dainty "Conservatory Ette," and a pas de deux that had music by Canned Heat and a psychedelic light show behind it.

Summer was over and time to go into my senior year in high school. I was ready to leave. I had enough of high school, and I was ready to start taking acting classes at junior college in Bremerton. They had a notoriously well-known acting teacher named William Harvey, known simply as Harvey, who had an outrageously FUN personality. He was a slender gay man, with jet black hair and a smile like a Chesire Cat.

CHAPTER THREE

JUNIOR COLLEGE AND RUNNING START

I had enough high school credits to only take three classes in the mornings, leaving my afternoons free. Another incredibly kismet thing was that Olympic Junior College was only two blocks away from my high school and I could just walk there after lunch and attend an afternoon acting class with Harvey.

We did basic sense memory exercises to begin with, and we were assigned to read *An Actor Prepares* by Constantine Stanislavsky, the father of Method acting from Russia. We did this for most of the first quarter, and then we were also invited to audition for the fall production of *Spoon River Anthology* by Edgar Lee Masters, a series of monologues taking place in a cemetery by the souls of the dead rising up out of their graves to tell you an encapsulated version of their lives.

I remember thinking "piece of cake" for the audition. I just have to talk and show emotion with what I am saying. I've been dancing in front of people most of my life, I can surely pull this off, right? Harvey assigns me a character to cold read, and we had to stand up in front of another twenty-five or so actors auditioning, watching us. WHAT A SHOCK!!! My mouth lost all its moisture, my heart was pounding out of my chest, and it's a fucking wonder I did not pass out. Nothing really came out the way I wanted it to, but somehow, I made it through and got to sit down. WHEW! As I was sitting there, I was thinking I would not get cast, how could I get a part, I SUCKED!

But to my amazement when we came to class the next day, I'd been cast along with twenty other classmates. Most of us got two different characters for the first and second acts. I cannot even remember my first character. It was something sort of bland, but my second character was about a young woman who gave birth to eight children and then pricked her finger on a rusty sowing needle and died young. Her last sentence was, "Sex is the curse of life!" which was funny since I was a virgin and so young looking.

I looked about thirteen, always young for my age. Anyway, the play was a hit. We had soldout houses and I was certainly hooked. I also loved being around a community of thespians who were artistic and likeminded, a wonderful, warm nurturing ambience. Bill Harvey was so very supportive, never ever sarcastic or mean, and a smart, good director, sitting at the back of the theater, smoking and taking notes. This was life changing for me, and definitely a step in the right direction, as I was beginning to think that I didn't want ballet as a career, although I kept taking classes weekly.

We started doing scene study with partners in class and I really enjoyed it. The winter plays were announced, a series of three one acts, and I was cast in two of them; the best being the silent film star, Pearl White, in Arthur Kopit's *Chamber Music.* It was basically about a women's insane asylum, with an all-female cast, each of whom thought they were a famous woman like Amelia Earhart or Gertrude Stein. It was a blast to perform, and my LLF Linda Kempski played Gertrude Stein.

My senior year in high school was a nonexistent joke. I had left the building for greener pastures, and it really turned out to be my favorite year living in Bremerton. While my senior classmates were at school whining about the fact that our class did not want a Senior Prom dance (if they had voted to have it, the theme would've been "Bullshit") per our class president and his council, I was at Olympic College starring as Ariel in Shakespeare's *The Tempest* and having the time of my life. The Bremerton Sun newspaper gave me the best review of all the actors, and it was the cherry on top of my acting experience with Harvey. Oh, and I suppose I should mention that I did receive the "Most Talented" award in our senior high school "Hall of Fame," and I did graduate cum laude.

CHAPTER FOUR

I DIDN'T CHOOSE SHOWBIZ, IT CHOSE ME!

At the beginning of my senior year, we were asked what our career goals were so we could start thinking of our next move towards it after graduation.

I'd already decided that being involved in professional entertainment was my goal, but NOT ballet. My actual goal was to be on TV and movies as a dancer-singer-actor, but it was surely not going to be achieved in Bremerton or even in Seattle.

I attended a ballet class once a week at a school in Tacoma that my grandma drove me to, across the scary Tacoma Narrows bridge. Margie was having health issues, and I still needed to advance, particularly my "pick up" skills, which were not fast enough.

The dance studio had a bulletin board with various forms of info about mostly dance, but one posted brochure caught my eye. It was for a performing arts college in San Diego called United States International University School of Performing Arts, featuring majors as Musical Theater performers. The brochure was well produced and well explained with pictures of its Dean, Jack Tygett, training some of his female dancers.

Auditions would be held in the Spring of 1971 to be accepted into the school, plus scholarships and financing available. DING DING DING DING DING!!! This was the ticket, my yellow brick road out of B-town to a kingdom called Hollywood.

Before seeing this brochure, I was like a ship without a sail, not knowing what to do to get to Southern California, to just go blindly trying to get work. It was WAAAAY too frightening for me to go from a town of fifty thousand to a city that had millions, and thousands of miles from home, family and friends.

Also, the instructors like Jack Tygett and his wife Marge were all previous show business professionals from TV, stage, and screen. Now this isn't necessarily a must for teachers to make you a pro, as it depends on the individual instructor, how much knowledge they impart to their students, but you DO need one or two who can tell you what is really going to happen when you get out into the real world as opposed to hearsay.

I had auditioned for the Joffrey Ballet and won another summer scholarship, which I partook of before going down to So Cal. As fate would have it, Edna McCrae took me aside towards the end of summer and told me that she and Bob (Joffrey) thought I was too sexy and would be better off pursuing another dance path, perhaps musical theater.

I trusted the opinion of professionals and told Edna I was already headed on that path. My personal life, other than really good fun friends, was not holding me back as well. After my first boyfriend, I had several other cute boys, including one who looked like Mick Jagger, who was my biggest celebrity crush, along with more boys in junior college, but none I wanted to make a future with.

I did talk one into deflowering me halfway through my senior year as I did not want to go to another college as a virgin. The guy happily assisted me with my wish, although I thought sex was surely overrated after that. I dodged a bullet, as neither of us used birth control, and actually with another beau after him, as I hadn't gone to planned parenthood to get fitted for a diaphragm yet.

Getting fitted for a diaphragm was a fun experience. I didn't want birth control pills or to even try them yet. I'd heard they made you gain weight and made you have mood swings, and I wanted neither at that time. When the attending GYN at planned parenthood folded the diaphragm with the jelly on it, it slipped out of her hand and went flying across the room, much to our delight and laughter. No wonder it had the title "flying saucer baby stopper" attached to it. Woo hoo!

CHAPTER FIVE

CALIFORNIA HERE I COME FOR THE NEXT TWELVE YEARS

I had to audition for USIUSPA to get accepted and to win a scholarship, so back to Cornish School of the Arts I went per usual, where it seems many a dance audition were held. It had a very large and airy main classroom and ballet barres on three sides of the room and the mirrors up front.

Unlike the other auditions that I'd gone to at Cornish, these were private at specific times, and we waited out in the hallway on benches until our names were called. I was told to prepare any songs, monologues, and memorized dances I had already learned, but some dancing would be given to us.

I was the only person out of about a half-dozen of us awaiting our turn in dance clothes, and I recognized no one that I was at SF Ballet and Joffrey with, hmmm? Later, I found out they were more from the singer/actor spectrum, and I was dancer/singer/actor.

After a brief wait, a dainty, pretty brunette woman stepped out wearing teacher's ballet attire and called my name as best she could (my last name of HOXIT has always been a challenge for most, it's Cherokee Scottish). She had a British accent, and introduced herself as Elaine Thomas, one of the ballet teachers on staff at SPA, and previously employed by Royal Ballet in London, cool!! She would be my auditioner.

I introduced myself, gave her a handwritten resumé, and proceeded to follow her into the classroom. First, she gave me a short ballet barre as a warmup and then gave me some center floor combinations. I did a jazz dance Margie Speck had choreographed, a Bojangles Robinson tap dance, and a monologue that I learned from doing Ariel in *The Tempest*, and the one solo song I sang as Ariel from the same. I wasn't at all nervous, as Elaine had a smiling face and happy vibe as she watched me and smoked her Virginia Slims cigarettes.

It's funny but many of my dance teachers and acting teachers (never vocal coaches) smoked in their classes at the time, which pretty much stopped by the 1990s. Many of us smoked, too, although I was a very light smoker, (two to six cigarettes a day), and never in the mornings. It made me sick. She said I did a good job, asked if all my contact information was accurate, and she hoped to be seeing me in San Diego come Fall. I'd receive my results via mail like most colleges, my acceptance or rejection letter. I believed I'd impressed her sufficiently, and indeed I did.

Sure 'nuf, about two weeks later, I not only received my acceptance letter, but I was offered a two-thirds ride scholarship as a musical theater dancer/singer/actor major for a full year. Room and board would not be free, but I could take out a low-cost student loan with a low interest rate, as I did NOT want my grandparents to pay for that, and my mom just didn't have the money as she was still raising my sister and now half-brother, Stan. She had remarried for about a year and a half, but that union didn't last either and we were back with my grandparents again.

September came around and I flew down to San Diego and was picked up and taken to my dorm and assigned two roommates who I did not know, but who ended up being my friends and taking me with them to their families on school breaks, although I did get to go home at Christmas.

The dorm rooms were little cottages with two bedrooms on the sides of a communal living room, and a bathroom with a double sink. We had several pools on campus, as well, and of course laundry rooms and a large cafeteria we had to walk to on a trail.

Interestingly, The School of Performing Arts was in downtown San Diego, and these dorms were quite far away on Pomerado Road near Mira Mar Airforce Base. We had a bus that drove us back and forth from the dorm rooms to the performing arts campus building, a three-story building that seemed to be designed to perfection for our needs.

The first floor was a lobby with regular classrooms and staff offices with a large staircase going up the middle to the second floor, which had three large dance classrooms with lovely large windows with a large outdoor balcony overlooking 4th Avenue, where we could go outside and screw around and smoke cigarettes.

There were other small rehearsal rooms with a couple of pianos for private voice lessons, and just odd areas where some of our boys, mostly, would smoke cannabis between classes. There was one more set of stairs where the two large theaters were situated, that went from the second to the third floor: Theater East and Theater West, with attached dressing rooms. The bathrooms were located off the third-floor lobby.

But no, I'm not finished yet. There was the basement that had a set of stairs, as well as an elevator to the first floor lobby. The basement had the basement theater that held about sixty people with a rather slippery cement floor, used for some acting classes and mostly student produced shows like the M.A. programs thesis shows that were fun and cutting edge. Also, the cafeteria was downstairs, small but doable because of staggered class schedules, and then about another dozen soundproof rooms for the music students, and sometimes group voice classes. We had music majors as well.

This was all in a single building, mind you. It was logistically and awesomely perfect for the approximately 350 students that were in attendance. We not only had musical theater majors, but we had also a master's program for that. We had an actor's program, a ballet majors' program, a modern dance program, and a technical theater program for those men or women desiring a career in the backstage aspects of theater, i.e. sets and lighting design. It was a perfect storm for all of us to succeed, unless you did not take it seriously, which some did not, or they just weren't physically cut out for it.

The school had only been going since 1967, and it was Fall of '71. We had a large freshman class of about a dozen girls and sixteen boys came in as Freshman for the musical theater, dancer/singer program, and another fifteen or so for the new singer/dancer group.

There was OODLES of talent and one thing that was noticeably different was that we were in general a much better-looking group as well as more advanced than much of the returning group of women, and thankfully they were in a different class than we were. They also had an edgy toughness about them, or as one of my classmates put it "like a bunch of bull dykes in a dark alley." We were scared of them to a certain extent, as I'd never been around mean girls in high school, just the male bully types, but here were my mean girls now.

Luckily, we Frosh bonded fairly quickly and hung with each other. I loved all my classes except for my acting teacher who was a total dud, especially after having somebody as literate and energetic as Bill Harvey, who as it turned out was the best acting teacher of my career. My favorite instructor here was dialect coach, Dennis Turner, from England, that I would have the following year.

I was put into the advanced ballet class almost immediately by my mentor Elaine Thomas, even though I enjoyed taking from her with the ballet majors. It was taught by a Norwegian man Earling Sunde, from Royal Danish Ballet. Earling wasn't so pleased about that and pretty much ignored me as I was the ONLY musical theater student he was forced to accept. I was better than the vast majority of ballet majors and that irritated him.

Luckily for me, Macarena Gandarillas, our stunningly beautiful musical theater dancer, originally from Chile came in shortly after I did, and was a comfort to me. After only two weeks of classes, it was time to audition for the first musical of the year, *The Roar of the Greasepaint, the Smell of the Crowd*, by Anthony Newly and Leslie Bricusse.

It was a small cast and was about the poor classes of England and how tough life was on the poor working man, set in late 19th century England. The supporting cast included a group of street urchins, basically teenage homeless kids. Looking young, I was cast, much to my surprise, as I didn't have a prepared audition song yet, and sang "Happy Birthday," but it was good enough to get into the Urchin chorus.

This was only my second musical, and once again I was having a blast. Even if you were only in the supporting cast, you still got to use all your multi talents, singing, dancing, and acting. It was very mentally and physically enriching for me. We were a huge hit with San Diego audiences and sold out houses nightly for the run. The reviews said we had a professional patina to our show as we were fortunate enough to have Jack Tygett as chorographer, and Charles Vernon from England directing.

We had been entered in the *American College Theater Festival* competition, and were selected for the semifinals, in line to be one of the top ten plays or musicals onstage at The Kennedy Center, in Washington D.C.

We went up to UCLA in Los Angles along with about a dozen other semifinalists from colleges around the state. We didn't get to see the other competitors at all but were told we were the best by many. There was an awards ceremony and dinner where we were awarded 1st place with a paid trip to Washington D.C. One of our leads, Michael Byers, who played Cocky, also won the Irene Ryan Award for best actor, and when I went into the ladies' room after the awards presentation, Irene Ryan was there!!! She was much prettier than she appeared in the *Beverly Hillbillies*, and the first REAL celebrity I had ever seen or been close to. I had to phone home that night and tell my folks about it.

Now it was Spring of '72 and time to fly to D.C. to the Kennedy Center and perform the show there. I had also been doing some children's theater for SPA, performed on the weekends, or travelling to some of the local schools on the weekdays. I had wanted to do more acting roles but quickly learned that I was pretty much going to have to be cast in musical theater roles, as that is what my scholarship was for. My roommate's boyfriend, Alan Ames, was directing children's theater, so he cast me in his productions in acting roles, which does prove the old saying "It's who ya know"!

We flew to D.C. for a full five days and were put up in an elegant older hotel in Georgetown. We rehearsed the show our first full day there, and then we were given a full twenty-four hours to see the monuments, White House, etc. We went to the Lincoln Memorial at night, which was our favorite, and then we hit the bars in Georgetown, and went out drinking. The drinking age was 18, woo hoo!!!

But the next morning, a couple of us were too sick and hungover to make it to a dress rehearsal, and Mr. Tygett had to come and have a talk with us. We sobered up and were just fine for the main performance. There was no winner for this event. We opened the festival, as we were considered the crème de la crème. We got to stay one more day, and saw SMU do their fantastic production of *Oedipus*, and a visiting college theater group from Poland perform *Romeo and Juliet* in Polish, that was so good you could understand the entire story!

We were flying back to San Diego to finish the school year. I was bursting with National pride and love for my country. Just visiting the nation's capital, let alone perform at the Kennedy Center was a life-changing experience and honor I will never forget. A couple of weeks after we got home, the school gave us an awards ceremony where all the cast members went onstage one at a time and the University president, Gordon Hilker, presented us with our very heavy bronze award necklace of excellence from the Kennedy Center and took our photos receiving the award. I have it to this day hanging in my "Hall of Fame" celebrity hallway and am so fortunate for the entire experience.

CHAPTER SIX

SUMMER BREAK AND XOREGOS MODERN DANCE COMPANY

I had heard from a friend of mine living in San Franciso about auditions for a modern dance company called Xoregos, owned and choreographed by a wild and enthusiastic Greek American woman, Shela Xoregos. Even though I didn't honestly like the modern dance style all that much, she was a very charismatic, good vibe woman with a tremendous love of dance and vibrant energy, and I accepted the company position of seven dancers and got free classes all summer long. I could stay with my friend, and I always loved San Francisco. The company of dancers was very likeable, even though I never saw a single one of them again after that summer.

We did a Paul Taylor piece that I really enjoyed, and I was paired with the principal male dancer, John Charles Musagetes, to do a pas de deux called "Turning" to dramatic electronic music that Shela had choreographed, based on Franz Kafka's book "Metamorphosis" about a salesman that wakes up one morning as a human insect. It was angular, eclectic choreography and John Charles was a strong and dynamic partner to work with. The piece ends with me on him, back-to-back, as he sidesteps bent over offstage with both of us moving our arms and feet randomly like an insect stuck on its back. It was my favorite part.

At the end of the scheduled number of performances, John Charles and I were invited to perform "Turning" in Monterey on an outdoor stage. Modern dance at that time and still today was done completely barefoot and the stage was probably over 90-degrees. It was very painful. When I did a barefoot turn in the middle of the dance, the crease on the bottom of my left foot split open, and as we went off stage as the insects, blood was indeed running down my leg.

Fortunately, we did not have to go back out for bows. It was by far the most painful injury I ever had as a dancer. That was the end of my short-lived career as a professional modern dancer. I'd made enough money to buy school clothes at various San Fransico shops and fly back home to Seattle for a couple of weeks before the Fall semester started, and see my family and some friends, smoke some weed, drink some beer, and chill.

So back at the dorms and I am assigned to an area of the dorms and campus farther away and newer than the other dorm rooms, known as "Siberia." I liked it. My new roommates were different this year. and I was sooooo pleased.

My other two roommates had not made it to sophomore year, and I believe it was a blessing for them. One just wasn't into the whole dancing thing, and the other one had freaked out on drugs and was not the right body type for the profession.

I next got to be with two dancer/singer majors who I knew were like myself, and serious about our future careers and studies: Denise Esola and Macarena Gandarillas. Macarena spent a lot of time over at her boyfriend Don's apartment in town. He was the only really cute guy at our school. Don was also a mime, and he taught us in class how to do the wall with our hands and to fly a kite. He had studied with Marcel Marceau and would eventually go professional.

I had come into a small inheritance from my great Aunt Viola from Bremerton, and I bought my first used car, a '65 powder blue Ford Mustang, with a black convertible top, for $750. My friend from school, Barry Koeb, went with me to a beach neighborhood to check it out, as it made me nervous to purchase a used car by myself, but it was in decent shape.

The Fall/Winter musical that year was Cole Porter's *Kiss Me Kate*. I really wanted the role of Bianca but instead was cast opposite Alex Christopoulos as his "special face" dance partner, as I was little and light and easy for him to pick up and lift, not because I had a great face. Alex was very sexy and charismatic and was playing Petruchio, the starring male. We also did a big dance number to "Too Darn Hot" that was sexy and fun. It was a huge cast and sold-out run, as usual. Jack Tygett could do no wrong.

Then it was time for winter break, and I was invited to fly to Oahu, Hawaii by my best friend at that time, June Linden. Her mom and older sister had moved there and her older sister Margret, who ironically was Go Go dancing at a strip club in downtown Oahu, said she'd get me a job there for the two weeks I was there. She would even give me a costume, and I could stay with June and her mom. So, how could I say no, and I could use some of the inheritance money for the plane trip.

The Lollipop Bar, a gentlemen's entertainment club, was in the middle of downtown Oahu, on the main drag, Kalakaua Blvd. It had two bars and a front room with one stage about 8' by 8', and the back room had two smaller stages. The smaller stages were surrounded by small tables, with the larger tables at the back of the room that could seat about ten people. There was a fairly large dressing room in the back, but NOT makeup tables (you did that before you came to work). You had to change into your G-string and top with your sheer to the waist pantyhose that you rolled the top of into the G-string. You wore whatever high heels you could dance in; I had brought my flesh toned Capezio heels that worked nicely for me.

There was a list that you signed at the bar with your name on it, and it was your job to remember the dancer in front of you. Then you picked up your serving tray and your checks and pen and first headed out to the tables in your assigned area to get your drink orders.

When you saw the dancer in front of you, you'd put your tray on the end of the bar and get ready to mount the stage in the main room and dance. It was only about 16-inches high, and easy to step up to from the side after the other dancer moved around to the back room, and the other two stages.

You would change stages when the song stopped and follow the dancer in front of you. Then, after the third stage, we would get down, pick up our drink order, and the process would begin again. Whoever came up with this idea was pretty smart, and it went very smoothly. You could also do private table dances if requested for another $5.00 a dance when you weren't in the rotation, but NO lap dancing and NO touching. That was far, far off in the future.

We had a big burly doorman that also served as a sort of host who'd direct the customers (mostly well to do Japanese businessmen or other male tourists from around the globe) to their tables. Of course, the bouncer was a big sweetheart (aren't they all), who was there to protect us! There were approximately twelve girls working on any given night, and I think we started around 6pm and the last call was midnight. The great thing is we had our days free to go to the beach and do whatever we wanted.

I loved the Ala Moana Mall and went there to buy clothes with my girlfriend, June. I bought a lovely long tropical patterned summer dress, and a very very sexy hand crochet hot pants ensemble, that was fairly revealing, that would get me into trouble later. And of course, a new bikini!!!

The Go-Go dancing was an interesting, positive experience and probably the worst thing that happened to me was that I got in a fight with June's mother, the volatile Karen Redding, a Finnish woman, who was just the opposite of June's loveable, sweet Papa Joe.

Anyway, I needed to get out of the apartment, and another friend from West High School, Barbara "Barb" King let me crash in her studio apartment for the last few days I was there. She stayed with her boyfriend, which was very generous of her. She had an indoor miniature pet bunny that would sometimes hop across the bed at night when I was trying to sleep. It was a sweet bunny, and I was amazed at how it was housetrained and would only poop and pee on the newspaper around its bowl when it ate or drank.

One more thing about the Lollipop Club: None of the young women there were sex workers or prostitutes. You had the option of dancing topless, and some of the women with larger breasts did, but not Margret Voore and me. I had no boobs to speak of anyway. I did go on dates with a couple of guys that came into the club, but that was my choice and not for money.

Back at SPA no big production was happening, and I had a lot of interest in telling my Hawaii story and experiences. I was studying dialect with Dennis Turner from England, and I loved it. Dialects came easy to me, and I thrived. Every week we were given a different dialect to work on, a paragraph to memorize, and the character traits to morph the vowels and consonants to the country it was from.

I'd also started private singing lessons, as it was recommended for me to do so for my musical theater goals. I had the lovely Sarah Flemming for my voice teacher, who helped me attain my vibrato and work on my audition songs, one up-tempo and one ballad.

At the beginning of the Fall semester, our now sophomore class had lost about six dancer/singers, mostly women, and the upper classes had had graduations. So, we were condensed into one advanced jazz/musical theater dance class under the tutelage of Marge Tygett, Jack Tygett's fun, energetic wife who had also danced in movies like her husband. I had studied tap dance with Marge in her advanced class as she was the hoofer, not her husband. For the most part I felt connected more to Marge because of that fact, plus her dance style was more feminine than her husband's, as it should be.

Marge taught us a lot of ethnic style dances such as Balinese and Scottish sword dancing, Highland-style. But the beginning of Spring semester was musical theater style and we girls did a dramatic dance to "Can't Help Loving that Man of Mine" from *Showboat* that I felt very uncomfortable executing. I raised my hand and told Marge this, and she had us all take a seat on the classroom floor. She advised us to think of having an orgasm with our boyfriend when having sex with them, and mentally I gasped, and my eyes were probably wide as saucers.

I had no boyfriend, as I had dated a few of the boys at school but no one steady, and not much sex with any of them. I thought to myself, "What's an orgasm?" but I was pleased how she spoke to us like adult women instead of teenagers, which we still were.

Then she gave us some priceless advice which was, "You are going to have to take some jobs where you won't like the music or choreography, but you need to do so to make a living, not porn, not striptease, but various musicals, TV shows, etc., and when you are doing them, you NEVER complain to the choreographer or director about it. TAKE THE MONEY AND RUN!"

Then she had one of our dancers perform it for us who was really hitting it out of the park with LOTS of feeling and facial expression, who ironically was known as the 'screamer" around campus. She did have a steady boyfriend and did enjoy her orgasms for many to hear. I couldn't wait to have one!

I'm telling this story to any young person who has to act, sing or dance a piece that they don't like and how to deal with it, and it WILL HAPPEN to you. Probably the vast majority of jobs you get you will like and relate to, but like your method of acting teaches you, think of a similar situation to get the correct feeling coming out of you and then do the task given you.

Later, in the year, Marge gave us a sexy jazz combination where you brought your hands sensually up the sides of your legs, and I really let loose. I slapped the outside of my thighs and drug them up as it was more sensuous than not. One of our more conservative female dancers ran up to Marge at the front of the classroom and said aloud, "Linda's touching herself, Linda's touching herself," and Marge just said, "That's the feeling I want," and she had all the girls do it. I had come into my sensuality as a jazz dancer at that moment. Jazz is slang for SEX, don'cha know?

Now it's March 1973 at my performing arts college. It's an ever fluid situation and the Spring musical is *Celebration*, a newer musical on Broadway in 1969 by Tom Jones and Harvey Schmidt (who wrote *The Fantasicks*) that no one was very familiar with. My singing voice is coming along swimmingly, and I had a talk with Jack Tygett about getting even a small acting or singing role in it. I didn't say as much, but I felt like I wasn't being challenged enough, as one other very talented actress was being chosen for the roles that were our type, and I was growing rather frustrated with that.

I had moved steadily along with William Harvey at Olympic College, but here it was mostly just dance or chorus roles. So, Jack said he'd consider it. We had the auditions a few days later. I did a solid job, but when the cast list came out, I was chosen for NOTHING, not even chorus. WOW.

The school was all abuzz about Sacramento Music Circus holding auditions at the end of the month up in Hollywood at the Hollywood Masonic Temple. Nobody had gone up the year before but there were about twenty-five of us who wanted to go this year.

Sacramento Music Circus was the ONLY summer stock company on the entire West Coast at that time and highly sought after and desirable. I handwrote my resumé on lined paper and gave them a picture of a model that looked almost identical to me, that I ripped out of a magazine as I did not have a headshot yet. To this day, I cannot believe I pulled that off. They accepted it.

I hitched a ride up to Hollywood with a car full of other alumni. We were called into a large room with a sprung wood floor, and up at the front was a table with three middle aged gentlemen and one cute one that was probably in his

30s. It was the chorographer, Walter Painter, who wore a small, brimmed straw hat and held a non-lit cigar. He taught us all a dance combination along with the other people from the greater L.A. area. There were six counts of eight, the standard for most auditions. Then we were split into groups of about eight and one group at a time performed it. At the end, we stood in a straight single line down from two rows and were told either to stay or thank you meaning "Buh bye." I was nervous but did a good job and was kept. Most of my alumni were released, but my ride waited for me.

It was time to sing. They did have an accompanist there on piano who also played our dance music for us. I had my sheet music to "I'd Do Anything" from *Oliver!* which I'd memorized and performed in a very sweet manner. I was nervous, but managed to do a decent, on-pitch job.

We all had to sit and watch the other dancers sing before and after our respective audition pieces. It was nerve-wracking, but a learning experience as well. After the final one, we were all thanked and started to put on the clothes we wore over our dance clothes. As we were doing so, one of the gentlemen from the table, Russell Lewis, called my name and told me to come over to them.

He told me they were certain they wanted to hire me, and asked if I was available from the end of June through the beginning of August for all five shows? Was this really happening or just a dream? I said oh yes, I sure was and accepted on the spot. I didn't even have to go to a callback. I made sure my contact information was correct and left happy but in shock! As it turned out, I was the only one from SPA that was chosen that summer season, what karma!

Word got around very quickly at school and to Jack Tygett, who had egg all over his face. Our relationship was just never the same after that, but I'd also felt that I'd got everything out of the situation there that I could, and I was becoming stagnant.

One of the M.F.A. students who I liked, Dan O'Connor, was doing a brand-new musical currently on Broadway for his thesis project called *Grease* that was all the rage, about high schoolers in the 1950s and their various cliques, mostly degenerates versus the goodie two shoe types. It used nomenclature of the time and had great songs and dances.

He did not have the rights, but he'd gotten permission from the powers that be to do it for two performances on the big stage for a weekend, it just wouldn't be advertised to the public, but the rest of the school could attend free.

Dan knew I was leaving, and probably for good after what Jack Tygett did to me, not casting me in *Celebration*. Dan offered me the role of Patty Simcox, the baton-twirling cheerleader, the epitome of a goody two shoes but a huge flirt with the "greaser" bad boys.

I accepted and started working on my role by borrowing a baton from my college roommate, Denise Esola, who was the baton twirling champion of the state of California, yet another cosmic gift! She taught me basic twirling, and I could even throw it into the air and catch it. Denise was also in the show as were a lot of my friends at SPA, and we had a blast. It is and remains a popular musical to this day and the most fun of any I ever did.

Then another MFA student, Bob Hanley, asked me to be a member of his cast in his MFA thesis, a compilation of songs and dances from various patriotic musicals, titled, *Like It Is*, Bob's catch phrase around school. I'd have some speaking roles and a solo dance. Bob was from New York. He was very Italian looking, had a slight New York accent, and was very talented. He was very into all things Broadway, and his nickname was "Broadway Bob." There were about twelve of us in the cast, all the best of the school's singers and dancers. This show was also a blast, and it was my last one at SPA.

CHAPTER SEVEN

NO GOING BACK

I was one of the last people to leave the dorm in June of '73, as I didn't have my apartment yet in Sacramento. I packed up my little stereo and records, my one set of towels and sheets, and my clothes, and headed for San Jose all by myself, in my '65 Mustang with no air conditioning. I could stay with my cousin Mary Saidy and her husband for about five days. Next, Denise invited me to stay for a few more days with her and her parents at their home in the small town of Plymouth, California, until my apartment was ready in Sacramento.

Sacramento Circus gave us a short list of apartments we could rent, and I was the only chorus member who chose my apartment complex. I had a studio apartment with a murphy bed, but it had a pool! There was plenty of street parking and I liked the fact that I was the only one living there.

There was still a couple of weeks left before we began rehearsals for the first musical of the season, *Camelot*. I went over to the tent, yes, a real, large circus tent, with swamp coolers in it, to check it out and let the staff know that I arrived. I had found the local St. Vincent DePaul Store to buy a few cheap plates, glasses, a pot, a pan, a bowl or two, and utensils to cook with. I found the grocery store and bought some food. I was truly alone, on my own for the first time in my life, but I was not scared. There weren't nearly as many people around back then, and it felt quiet and safe.

A couple of days go by, and I'm starting to make my dinner, and I hear a knock at the door. It's producer Howard Young. He wanted to know if I would like to do the part of one of the Ugly Stepsisters in their children's theater production of *Cinderella*. It would pay an extra $25 for the week and give me something to do. I said sure and then asked him how long you boil corn on the cob, as that was what I was making with my hot dog. "About eight minutes," was his answer, and he took his leave.

The next day, I met six of the other chorus members who were all really nice and fun. We only performed *Cinderella* twice the following weekend to very small groups of young children, but I had lines and a harmony duet with Dorothy Nichols, who was the other Ugly Stepsister, but actually we were both quite cute!

Our summer lineup was a good selection of lively musicals with good characters and scores: *Camelot, Cabaret, Hello, Dolly! Oliver! and Applause*. At that time, all the casting was done out of Los Angeles, except for a few walk-on bit parts to thrill the locals. All of the leads and principals were celebrities from TV and movies, as were supporting roles, and we got excited at the start of every show to meet them, as this was also our first AEA (Actors Equity) union show. We all had to join AEA and were put on a budget to do so. We had increments taken out of our $200 weekly paycheck until the $300 was paid off.

Now, up until this point in time I had only LIKED musical theatre but when I did *Camelot*, I fell in love with it. It starred John Raitt, Harve Presnell, and the beautiful Susan Cabot as Guinevere. This was the most magical summer of my life.

When we rehearsed, we had to learn the four main aisles of the theatre first, as everything revolved around them. They were at about a 25-degree slope that went down to the round, revolving stage. This was theater in the round, which I had never done before. We would use the aisles to enter and exit, but also to sing in groups, highlighted with a spotlight on us. This was an enhancement to the entire performance experience, with the audience right next to us, and they loved it. They were so close, they could reach out and touch us, but they behaved themselves and never broke the fourth wall.

By this time, the most hilarious story we heard came from Erica Young, producer Howard Young's daughter, who was head of the wardrobe department at that time. As the story goes, Harve Presnell was being fitted for his Lancelot tunic. As she was hemming the bottom of it, he requested it to be an inch or two higher, "for the ladies." So, she complied and then he got "wood." He wasn't a harasser, but he did do a lot of making eye contact with the chorus women and smiling, so we nicknamed him "Horny Harve."

Opening night rolled around and I was not nervous for the first AEA show of my career. After the emotional jousting song, the entire chorus of sixteen of us exited up an aisle, led by the men of our chorus in their robes, some with long hair flowing behind them, carrying swords or jousting lances, and it made me catch my breath seeing it. We WERE in Camelot!

Next came "The Lusty Month of May" and Guinevere was put on a swing with flower covered ropes that swung back and forth across the stage. My darling dance partner Michael Eselun and myself were on the side she swung towards, and another couple pushed her from behind towards us across the stage. It was her solo, "Tra-la, it's May," which she sang joyfully, but about the third or fourth verse, in she came swinging at us, only mouthing the words, as she had forgotten the lyrics. It only lasted two short verses, but Michael and I looked at each other with eyes like saucers and hearts in our throats. She did recover, and I don't think the audience even noticed.

Every musical had a run of only a week, seven performances, Monday through Sunday. During the day, we rehearsed the following week's musical, as there were no matinees. We were ALL concerned whether we could do one musical while learning the next one, but somehow our brains adapted.

There were lovely programs the audience could purchase, and the cast was given one free at the end of every show which we timidly asked the stars to autograph. Harve signed mine "To the prettiest courtesan of all," and I did find it amusing.

Musical number two was *Cabaret,* and I was excited about it, with its great score. The big star playing Sally Bowles was Jessica Walters of *Play Misty for Me* fame. She did a decent job singing the songs, but she was no Liza Minnelli. I was a Kit Kat Club girl, and we got to do "Don't Tell Mama," singing and dancing with Jessica.

I was placed next to her for that number, and she had Walter Painter move me to the outside of the line away from her as she said aloud, "Linda is too good looking to dance next to," but she said it in a nice way, and I didn't mind. I liked Jessica. She was fun and mischievous. If anything, I was just a much better dancer than she was. I was disappointed that we were not going to perform "Mein Herr" on stools like in the movie a la Fosse, but perhaps it was too sexual for Sacramento at that time.

On opening nights, we had no cast party provided by Lewis & Young. We did receive a glass of champagne back in the subscriber's patio area, if we wanted it. It was my first champagne other than some cheap rotgut fizzy wine I'd had as a teenager in Bremerton. But on this opening night, one of the stagehands posted on the bulletin board, a party at their funky midtown Sacramento house and BYOB, so I decided to go.

Much to my amazement, Jessica went. I found a place near her, and she was smoking which I also did at the time, and she was smoking my brand, Virginia Slims! So, we talked about how we controlled how much a day, and when we smoked. I believe she said she was up to six a day, but I was only smoking two a day, unless I went to a party or bar and drank.

I also couldn't afford more than a pack a week, but once again, I never smoked with my coffee in the morning like so many. Then several of us asked her about *Play Misty for Me*, playing such a crazed woman. She said she just dug deep into herself and decided to play it more like a crazy MAN. She showed us how she held the knife up to stab Clint Eastwood and twisted her wrist around like a man would, to get a harder thrust downward. I found it fascinating. I will never forget her showing us that.

Musical number three was *Hello, Dolly!* Now here comes the fun again. Dolly was Jo Ann Worley from *Laugh-In* and Vandegelder was Jesse White, the "Maytag Man" from the Maytag washing machine commercials. Who says you can't get famous from commercials? Minnie Fay was played by Nancy Fox from the TV series *Temperatures Rising*, and many years down the road we'd be on Broadway together in another musical. Then there was movie star Gloria DeHaven as Irene Malloy, singing "Ribbons Down My Back" with a heavenly soprano voice. What a cast!

The rehearsals were a blast—Jo Ann and her loud voice and raucous laugh, are you kidding me? The musical had a great score and tons of dancing, in fact there was a song called "Dancing," and we got to do jete's in a big circle led by Nancy Fox. "Put On Your Sunday Clothes," dressed in late 19th century ruffled finest with parasols was such a happy number, and of course there was the "Waiter's Gallop," with just our men, but it always brought the house down and still does. I've only seen *Dolly!* a few times since but no other woman playing that character EVER compared to Jo Ann Worley, not even close.

Musical number four was *Oliver!* And this musical was the most unusual casting I'd ever seen or experienced. Nancy, the abused lead female was played by African American dancer/singer Paula Kelly of *Sweet Charity* the movie fame. Fagin was played by none other than Leonard Nimoy. The actor playing Bill opposite Paula was no one of note, and Paula was such a strong actress and singer, she ran all over him, but he was a white man, my first ever color-blind casting experience and it worked for me.

We were taught immediately on the first day of rehearsal to basically leave the stars alone, unless of course, you had a scene with them, or they spoke first. No real groveling for pictures or autographs, so everybody left Leonard Nimoy alone.

But one day watching him rehearse on stage, I realized for the first time that some of the so called "stars" were there because of that, and not their amazing talent. Leonard played Fagin looking down into the stage, sort of hunched over, and he was hard to hear as he sang "You've Got to Pick a Pocket or Two." It was very unimpressive and hard to believe that director Jack Bunch didn't make him get his performance up and out to the audience.

The actor playing the Artful Dodger was Stuart Getz, a cute young actor who'd been on some TV shows and was fun to work with. Stuart was red haired with freckles and an impish face. He was around the age of our chorus, fun to hang out with, and livened up the otherwise low-key scenes with Leonard Nimoy's Fagin. But other than singing a drinking song with Paula every night and acting like a drunk wench, there was almost no dancing and not much for the chorus to do, but you know, take the money and run, right?

Musical number five was *Applause*, and was fresh off of Broadway, our newest and most modern musical. Our big stars were "No Nose" Nanette Fabray, who'd had so many nose jobs her nose looked like two nostrils and was a continual fascination to me, and Kathleen Nolan, her nemesis in the show, from the TV series, *The Real McCoys*.

The musical, based on *All About Eve*, was about two female divas on Broadway vying for the same roles. The rest of us were the gypsies, the dancers and singers who worked on Broadway shows as chorus and went from show to show trying to get a break and get better roles, basically playing ourselves.

The provocative Barbara Luna was hired to play Bonnie, who was the leader of the gypsies, and to be Walter Painter's assistant choreographer. She was the sexiest, most erotic woman I'd ever seen in my life. The way she styled herself was simply outstanding with tight jazz clothes that exposed a very flat, bare stomach enhanced by midriff half leotards, and a gold belly chain. It was interesting to the rest of us that Walter had not had an assistant all summer until this time. Hmm?

We got to wear our own clothes that were as provocative as we had, with the help of whatever Erica Young could come up with. One of our female singers was put in a bondage outfit with a whip for one of the party numbers. I was put in Daisy Duke shorts with a macrame top and my blue suede knee high boots, but then a very gross blonde afro wig to minimize my real looks, as they did not want me to compete with the leading ladies.

We had a great time with this, our final musical of the summer, and Lewis and Young told us all that we were hired back for next summer if we would like to work the summer of '74. They said that we were unequivocally the best chorus they'd had since Music Circus started back in 1951. Wow.

Also, Walter Painter said he would hire me for projects in L.A. as well, and I sure needed the work as I was not going back to USIUSPA. I think Walter and I had a crush on each other, but he was married to Charlene Painter, a professional dancer, wasn't he?

What is my next career choice? Certainly not back to Bremerton or Seattle, so Hollywood here I come. Another male cast member from the chorus wanted to move from his hometown of San Jose to Los Angles, too, and he suggested we get a two-bedroom place together. I thought, well fine. A bunch of our chorus cast had been sharing a large old house for the summer, male and female, and at that point he was my only option. People from the chorus already lived and had places there, or some were not going to move at this time, so let's go for it!

CHAPTER EIGHT

HELLO HOLLYWOOD HELLO

So, my chorus friend—let's just call him Dick—and I loaded up our respective cars and headed on down to L.A. We both had our own set of friends we could couch surf on for a couple of days while we met for coffee in the morning and went searching for an apartment.

It only took us two days to find one that was suitable, but also one we could both afford, as we had limited funds. I always think of the saying "$600 and a mule" because that was the amount slaves were supposedly given after the Civil War to get a fresh start as free men. I had "$600 and my '65 Mustang", and at least sheets, towels, cookware, and plates. So did Dick, but neither of us had furniture, so we had to also find a furnished place.

What we acquired was rather frightening, looking back on the situation. It was in East Hollywood across Vine Street, kitty corner from the Hollywood Ranch Market, on a cross street I simply do not remember the name of.

This was Fall of 1973, and that neighborhood was rather run down and dicey. The building had a high fence and a lobby with a manager who lived onsite that you had to ingress and egress out of. The apartments inside were made of smooth stucco and the courtyard was somewhat rundown, but you could tell at one time it'd been lush and tropical.

The apartments made a semicircle around the courtyard and most were one bedrooms or studios. Ours was the biggest one with stairs that went up to the second story, two bedrooms, a large living room, one bathroom and a small kitchen. There were only queen-size mattresses on the bedroom floors and no frames, but we were okay with that, and they were clean and unstained. We had a table and chairs and a small couch. It was all clean, and what we could afford.

We put the required down payment down and moved in. We were told by the manager that Rudolf Valentino and other silent film stars once lived there, and if you'd seen the art deco style, it seemed entirely possible. It was built in 1920, and it did have a floral smell, as well. As the first couple of weeks moved on, we saw that our apartment neighbors were old, sad-looking retired men, but very benign. The street, however, seemed to have a considerable amount of criminal activity going on, with sirens and apparent thefts happening a couple of times a week.

We did get a phone, but we had no TV. We would walk across the street in the mornings to do our marketing and buy one or both trade papers, *The Hollywood Reporter* and/or *Variety*, to look for auditions. Neither of us had any agents yet, and back then, even if you did, many auditions for dancers and singers did not require agents. The ads posted a specific type, i.e. age, gender, ethnic background, and sometimes height, never weight, and the talent style they were looking to hire, also age, location and address.

Looking back on this whole new chapter of my life in Los Angles, I am amazed at my bravery of going from a smallish, almost crime-free city to the relative safety of living in college dorms on a college campus, to moving to the second largest city in the entire U.S. I was learning where I was going and driving there, too, and not getting robbed or molested, as I was very young-looking for my age. I definitely had guardian angels looking over me! I was extremely driven to make it in show biz, what I'd trained tirelessly to achieve for the past decade.

Things were progressing nicely, although there was no new job yet. I was going to auditions constantly, grabbing a dance class here and there from Bobby Banas, who I was told to study with by the Tygett's, and generally enjoying being a professional union entertainer now.

A fellow who I'd dated for a short period of time at the end of my engagement with the Xoregos Dance Company in San Francisco, named Norman, heard I had moved to L.A. He was the lead singer in one of those rock bands that played cover tunes in Holiday and Ramada Inns, traveling around the state. He wanted to come and see me. So, heck yeah, he was a cute, nice guy. We went out for a burger and then back to my apartment for a little tete a tete, as we were alone. But then Dick came home. Normon and I were sitting close together on the couch, and I could tell immediately Dick was not pleased. I felt a vibe you could cut with a knife.

Well, Norman had to leave anyway and go to band practice, so he split. I asked Dick what was up, and he said, "I thought we weren't going to see other people while living together?"

I was shocked. Nothing of the kind had ever been discussed or agreed upon. I then realized Dick had other plans for our relationship, even though I had never as much been asked out by him the entire summer in Sacramento. Living together was NOT going to work. I had no desire for any sort of romantic relationship with him, as he simply was not my type. So, I said, "I'm going to have to ask that you find someplace else to live, as I don't want any sort of intimate relationship. It's almost the end of the month so please start looking. You've got five days". Now that may sound harsh, but he had lied to me about his actual motives for wanting to live with me, and he knew this was only fair, so he grudgingly complied.

Now I needed another roommate to take his place, and for sure this time another female. The next day I headed to both of the dance studios I was taking from at the time and searched their bulletin boards for other female dancers looking for roommates and there I found Brantly Bright—what a wonderful stage name she had! I gave her a call, and she came over that afternoon.

I gave her a brief description of the situation, but ironically, she was staying with another young woman in one of the smaller apartments in our complex. What were the odds of that? And THEY weren't getting along, their place was sooooo small. So, she said yes immediately and was able to wait until Dick left a few days later.

And still another bizarre coincidence was that Brantly had come down from San Francisco where she'd been a member of San Francisco's corps de ballet. Fucking WOW! Now of course, I'd never made it into their company, not even close, but we had that in common and knew some of the same dancers and teachers.

Brantly was a beautiful young woman, my age, with milky white skin, brunette hair, and huge eyes, plus the svelte, toned ballet body. As far as I could tell, she'd come to Hollywood seeking more than a ballet career, especially with her great looks. I don't mean to be mean here but many a ballet dancer was not always the best-looking female. San Francsico did have the better-looking women as far as the company went. Her background was all ballet, and she didn't sing or act or do other dance forms like tap and jazz, and Los Angles was NOT a ballet town.

We got along swell and she started dating a very sexy, handsome photographer, Tony Lowe, who had a hidden loft- style apartment right underneath ours. The way it was constructed you could barely tell it was there. He had a back door that opened to our street. We met him one day, with his curly black hair and a pirate smile. He and Brantly hit it off immediately, and she stayed with me, but spent most of her time with Tony, lucky her.

So shortly after I met Brantly as a roommate, there was an ad in the trades for young female dancers, petite young women who could sing, 5'4" or thereabouts, but no taller. Well, I was 5'3", and didn't that just sound perfect? I'd been auditioning for a month with no luck yet. It was from 10am-3pm at the Century Plaza Hotel in Century City, Room 120 on the 12th floor. You'd have to sing, no dancing yet. Alrighty then.

CHAPTER NINE

RAY ANTHONY AND HIS BOOKEND REVUE

Here ... I am taking a deep breath and a slow exhale as this will be my most difficult chapter to write and relive. As I've been writing this, I have been reliving, revisualizing my memories as I'm sure most people experience who write their memoirs do, almost the main reason to put in the time, and the effort to do so.

This is certainly the most unfortunate memory and possibly what parents have nightmares about happening to their pretty, young daughters who move thousands of miles from home to dirty, sinful Hollywood.

Legend has it that the likes of Clara Bow, Marilyn Monroe, Shirley MacLaine, et al, experienced the trend of powerful men in Hollywood expecting sexual favors from starlets on the way up. In truth, they really were not all like that, and in fact most were more like father figures to me. None of my college professors or Lewis & Young of Music Circus ever sexually aggressed me—in fact, NO MAN had ever been forceful with me.

Back to this audition. I had dressed up in my cutest hot pants outfit as this was just a singing audition. I had my sheet music and resumé with me and this time my resumé was typeset and I had copies made by a printer on Hollywood Blvd. I also had copies of a headshot that was actually me. I was such a young professional now! The ad in the trades said it was for a well-known band, so I thought maybe a rock band, how fun would that be?

Century City was easy to get to, and the Century Plaza Hotel still looked new and swanky. In fact, all of Century City was pristine and clean compared to Hollywood at that time, which was fairly disgusting and filthy. The hotel had a big parking lot behind it, so I parked and made my way in the huge, modern lobby. I went up the elevator to the 12th floor and followed a sign that said audition for singers, Room 120 this way, with an arrow pointing to the right. It was a fairly long hallway with many rooms, but this one was all the way to the end of the hall, in fact, the last one, next to a stairwell.

The hotel room door to 120 was wide open and inside sat a single man. He was very very tan, but he looked like he had some sort of spray tan on as well. His hair was jet black and he was sitting behind a small table. He rose and asked me if I was there for the audition, and I smiled and said yes. He was on the short side, about 5'8".

He introduced himself as bandleader Ray Anthony, and asked was I familiar with him and his band? I said I was not, but looking at him I imagined that his band was probably like Lawrence Welk on his TV show. I introduced myself and he had me take a chair at the table opposite him.

He was smiling a lot at me with his gleaming Hollywood smile and his dark, slightly beady eyes. He wasn't bad looking I thought, somewhere between 40 and 50, hard to tell with that deep tan. I was 20, so he was about the same age as my dad. I gave him my resume which he looked over and seemed pleased with and asked me what my vocal range was. "Alto, and fairly strong," I said. "I've done mostly musicals, as you can see, so I can belt." Then he explained what I was auditioning for.

"I have a group of dancer/singers called "The Bookends" that travel with me and my band of ten men," he said. "They dance and sing modern songs and older songs from the 1940s big band era, and dances from that period, as well. I use four gals, but one just quit, and another one is leaving at the end of the year, as she's pursuing other interests here in L.A. We have bookings scheduled for Acapulco, Chicago, and Evansville, Indiana for the next four months. So really, I'm actually just going to hire one new gal, but I'll be choosing two for L.A.'s run, capiche?"

That sounds so interesting and fun! So YES, where do I sign up?

"Well, first you've got to sing for me," he said.

I gave him my sheet music, but unlike other auditions, there was no accompanist in the room at a piano.

"Just stand and sing for me acapella." My audition song at the time was "I'd Do Anything" from the musical *Oliver!* It was simple to do, and I sang it in a very sweet, friendly manner. I was pitch perfect and animated. I nailed it.

So, Ray said, "Can you start rehearsing this week? I'll pay you $100 a week and if you go on the road and I choose you, it'll go up to $250, plus rooms and travel paid for."

"ABSOLUTELY," was my enthusiastic reply.

Then he said, "And why don't you come back for dinner tonight and we can discuss the job more."

Dinner, like from a restaurant? My brain was doing a little dance. When was the last time I'd been invited to ANY dinner, maybe a year ago on a date at school? Hell, yes, what time?

"Oh, about 6pm, and meet me up here again and we'll go," he replied.

Alrighty then, a new paying job and a decent meal. I'd been eating a lot of yellow squash, hamburger and Top Ramen, as I wasn't much of a cook yet either, though I did cook some growing up. It was the middle of the day, so I went back to the apartment and told Brantly about my new job, bursting with excitement. Brantly was not having much success finding work either, although she did have some beautiful new headshots, thanks to her boyfriend Tony Lowe, who was a professional rock and roll photographer.

I drove back to the Century Plaza Hotel and went back up to Ray's room. This time the door was closed and when I knocked Ray asked me to come in. I noticed he was dressed somewhat more casually. The small table that had been toward the far side of the room was now at the foot of the bed with a chair on either side. Then he told me we were going to have room service, as they had a great room service menu from the main restaurant in the hotel. There was also a bucket with ice and a champagne bottle chilling in it by the side of the table.

Well, okay, I'd never had room service, just seen it on TV and in movies. He gave me the menu and had me sit down opposite him. He recommended the filet and said he was having that, too, so sure. He popped the champagne and poured a glass each and we toasted to my new job as we waited for room service.

I told him my background and that I was far from my home in Washington State. He told me I'd like the other girls, that they were really cute and fun. Then he asked if I had a boyfriend, and more small talk.

The food came and it was great. It also had a broiled tomato half with parmesan cheese and a baked potato, wowzah! I had just put the last bite of my dinner in my mouth and took a sip of champagne, when he came around the table and literally picked me up and threw me on the bed. For a little man he was strong. The hotpants outfit that I still had on was easily and quickly removed, and then he ...

And now I stop because it's the year 2025 and he's still alive with dementia at 103 and people would say that I'm being cruel, as he cannot defend himself and besides it's always "He said she said." But I'm sure you'll read between the lines.

I was damned mad and put my clothes on, grabbed my purse, and left without saying much, although he seemed pleased with himself. As I drove home, I thought that I probably wouldn't hear from him again, I probably lost my new job, but at least I was NOT traumatized, not crying. It was good to be angry. I would not tell Brantly or ANYBODY what had transpired for years, I just said he had tried to force himself on me, but I got away.

It wasn't until the #Me Too movement became strong in 2017, when all of the Harvey Weinstein and Bill Cosby allegations came out that I finally admitted what had happened, I didn't even tell the other Bookends when I started working with them two days later. Turns out he didn't fire me and had his secretary Jean Plant call me to begin rehearsals. He needed me as much as I needed the job. I just wouldn't ever be alone with him in a hotel room again, or any strange man ever ever, ever again.

Rehearsals were held on the stage of the Westside Room, where we'd be performing. I walked in the first day and there in front of me were five of the cutest, best dressed young women I'd ever seen. Some were really sophisticated and smoked Nat Sherman cigarettes they held in their manicured hands. One of them would be my friend for years to come. She was Charkie Phillips, who was paid to teach me and the other recruit, Cozette, the choreography.

Ray would come in with his trumpet later with our organ player and work on the songs with us in the afternoon. It was a small stage, and we had limited room for the dances. For the songs, our microphones were all set together.

The gals he'd hired were strong dancers more so than singers, and he wanted to do more and difficult dances for the tour. None of the other Bookends were taking class except me, so Ray asked for a professional choreographer, and I recommended Bobby Banas. Bobby came in and set three new dances with us. When I think about the fact that I got Bobby a job, it blows my mind. He'd been one of the best dancers in movies and TV shows of the 60s, and little me got him a job.

The dance routines that Bobby choreographed were very fast and difficult. Edgar Winters' "Frankenstein" just kicked ass. We also did "The Bunny Hop" with an extended instrumental version because Ray had written that and it was a big hit for him. Those two dance routines were added later but first Cozette and I had a week to learn the existing show. It wasn't that difficult.

There was an opening number to "Get Ready Cause Here I Come," a backup vocal routine to "You've Got a Friend" with Ray singing lead, a medley of World War II-era songs in four-part harmony, "Juke Box Saturday Night" into "Flat Foot Floogie" into "Bei Mir Bis Du Schön" back into "Juke Box Saturday Night" then into jitterbugging with each other.

Later we did "Superfly" as spies with trench coats on, a vocal rendition of "Boogie Woogie Bugle Boy," and the finale, "When the Saints come Marching In." Whew! I struggled with my low contralto part and Ray would walk over to me sometimes and play my beginning note in my ear, and after that I was fine. Cozette and I were asked to stay and watch the show, and it was just fucking darling, and so were the Bookends.

As rehearsal time went on, Cozette and I were filled in about Ray "Agony" as he was referred to behind his back by the girls and his band. As a small child, Ray had been forced to learn and play trumpet by his overbearing Italian father, who had some sort of band—their last name was really Antonini. If Ray didn't practice enough, he was locked in a dark closet and forced to practice for a couple of hours.

He was hired at a young age to play with the Glenn Miller Orchestra, and as of this date, April 2025, he is the only living member of that group. After a couple of years, he broke away from Glenn Miller and formed his own band named after himself. He WAS ambitious.

He wrote "The Bunny Hop" and had hit recordings of "Harbor Lights" the theme from *Dragnet*, the theme from *Peter Gunn*, and others. He also did some movies playing himself with the Glenn Miller Orchestra or his own band, notably *The Girl Can't Help It* starring Jayne Mansfield, and *High School Confidential*, starring his soon to become his only wife, Mamie Van Doren. They were two large- breasted women in the vein of Marilyn Monroe, with sexy faces and blonde bombshell hair. He was considered a hot man and people referred to him as the poor man's Cary Grant, desired by many women of my mom and grandma's age, but not by me.

At this time, Ray was building a new house in the Hollywood Hills that wouldn't be finished for a couple of years, so he made a deal for himself to live at the Century Plaza Hotel for the run of the show. The girls had a room of their own on the 10th floor where they could also hang out, put on make-up, and even take a nap if needed.

Ray Anthony and his Bookend Revue had just opened one week prior to the posted audition in *Variety*. On opening night, he and another Bookend were in an elevator on the way down to the stage and dressing rooms. The minute the elevator door closed, he started to try and kiss and molest her, even though she tried to shove him off. When the elevator hit the first floor, she told Ray, "That's it, I quit," and went back up to the Bookend room on the 10th floor, got her stuff, and left, leaving only three Bookends on opening night!

Oh, I know her name, and I met her many times at various places after this happened, but I won't be divulging some of the real names in my stories to protect reputations. But when I heard this story, she became my Bookend hero for doing this!

Yet another Bookend had a deal of quid pro quo verbally worked out with Ray. She was a gorgeous gal, but struggled with her weight, which I always thought was not that bad. She was voluptuous, and her extra pounds were in all the right places. Still, Ray held this over her head, so twice a week after the show, she had to go up to Ray's room and have sex to keep her job. She was open with all of us about the situation and I thought that was brave of her. But boy was I beginning to get a vivid picture of who my new boss was. The one Bookend leaving after the '73 holidays was Candy Darlene Valentine, who'd been one of his main Bookends for several years, and probably had the best vocal chops of all of us. She was also very pretty, animated, and hilarious. She would be the one that Cozette and I would be chosen to replace, as confusing as all this is.

I did very well learning the show. I was one of the better dancers, but I did struggle, as I said, with the four-part harmony. But with this experience I did learn how to do it and not cheat with the melody, like I had in previous singing situations. I was pleasant to Ray but stayed away from him as much as possible. He knew I was wary of him and wanted no more physical contact.

I also learned that his marriage to sex-kitten actress Mamie Van Doren had failed, and he was very single now. Rumor had it that Ray would come home from work and find Mamie in bed with other men, and Ray couldn't take that. They did manage to have one son, Perry, who came to see our show a couple of times. He came with Ray's really nice brother, Leo, who was a clarinet player in Ray's band. Perry was about 10 years old, had special needs, and I felt sorry for the poor kid.

I enjoyed the show, and I enjoyed the other Bookends, who were funny and so cute. Ray also made us wear wigs even though some of us, including myself, had great hair. We also wore false eyelashes and padded bras, except for the one voluptuous Bookend, as she did not need the padding! I certainly needed the padding.

When we arrived for a show, usually in our jeans, Ray insisted that we go up to our Bookend room and change into floor-length gowns before making our way through the hotel to our dressing room. He wanted us all to look like Mamie Van Doren-style movie stars, in his own words.

So, three months passed, and the show would be going on the road to Acapulco, Chicago, and Indiana for four months. It was time for Ray to choose between myself and Cozette. We both had done good jobs. I had managed to not be alone with Ray, and he hadn't called me and invited me to his room, thank God!

But the first week of December, he called me into his dressing room before the show and said "Okay, here's the deal: You can do what (overweight girl) is doing, or I'll choose Cozette."

I said, "I am not interested in doing 'that,' plain and simple." So, he said, "Well you're dancing isn't up to par anyway," since I had to have a reason to tell unemployment, and it couldn't be because I wouldn't have sex with him, of course.

I walked out of his dressing room and back to our room and Cozette was called into his room so he could tell her she got the job. He did not want sex from her. I told the others what transpired, and they were incredulous, especially that he criticized my dancing. He could have gone for my struggle with harmonies. I was mad, but at least I'd get unemployment, which I couldn't get after working just six weeks in Sacramento.

A week went by, and I started to look for more auditions, and then on my night off, as I still had two weeks left, the phone rang. It was Ray and he sounded very sweet, unusually so. Then he says, "(Voluptuous girl) decided she doesn't want to go on tour, so how would you like to take her place? (The truth was she told him she would not continue in their relationship anymore.) I queried, "What kind of trick is this? I am not interested in a sexual relationship."

"No trick," he said, "you know the show, with the new dance routines and all." I paused for a few seconds and replied, "Yes, I'd love to continue doing the show, but if you try anything funny, I'll get on a plane and leave, capiche? No calls or requests to see you, or go on a date, I only work for you as a Bookend."

"OK you got it, it's a deal, see you at work."

I hung up and did a happy dance. I had him over a barrel. So, I told Brantly, and she wanted to move in with Tony now anyway. I had a friend who had a parking space in a building where I could keep my car. I packed all my stuff in the trunk and embarked on my first road job.

CHAPTER TEN

ACAPULCO, THE PLAYBOY CLUB CHICAGO AND BEYOND

I'd never been in Mexico, the closest being San Diego, and Acapulco was quite the way to start. We were playing the showroom at the Acapulco Princess Hotel that was actually outside the city of Acapulco, around the bay of Puerto Marques.

Boy what a stunning resort! It had about 300 rooms, several restaurants, and a gourmet dining room where we were invited by Ray for a meal that started off with turtle soup! There was a pool bar with waterfalls, and the Pacific Ocean and beach if you wanted that. We stayed away from that as we were told the "banditos" hung out there. There was a basement disco that we made good and frequent use of.

We went into town for shopping and there was a fabulous boutique there called Piasa's, owned by a dashing man who was the designer/owner. Affectionately known as Papa Piasa, he was in his late 30s. We dated from time to time.

He had a jungle cabin and a parrot, and we went there once on my day off and dropped windowpane acid. The best trip of my life and the final one. The tropical vegetation was neon green, the flowers neon pink and red, the parrot (yes, parrot) neon blue. I hadn't taken LSD since Bremerton, four years before.

I also dated a handsome Brazilian man who took me water skiing for hours at Puerto Marques, where there were many huge manna rays, although we saw none. We only did shows at night, so we had oodles of free time in the day. We had to do a certain number of activities with Ray as we were his celebrity Bookends. We got invited to a couple of very glamorous high-end parties at Armando's, a nightclub and disco. There was one very funky party in a weird jungle-style large hut with dirt floors. It was our day off, and we were pissed we had to spend it with Ray. I had to use the restroom, and it was very filthy, but I had to go bad, and I sat down on a toilet with no seat cover protection. Uh oh.

Sure enough, a few days later, Charkie and I smoked part of a joint—the weed was plentiful there. When I was putting my underwear on, I saw little bugs crawling in my pubic hair. OMG, and I was stoned on top of it. I told Charkie, "I think I have crabs," although I'd never seen or had them before.

The Princess had a resident doctor who was free to the clientele and us, so the gals suggested I go and see him. He had an office right there in the basement of the hotel, and sure 'nuf he diagnosed them. He gave me some topical cream and also told me to shave all my pubic hair and put the cream on until they were gone for several days and also wash all my underwear AND all my clothes as well.

So, I went back upstairs to my room and got in the bathtub and shaved my bush off with the other Bookends watching. I was still stoned and crying as they watched me and teased me. NONE of them got them either, just me! They were gone for good in about three days.

I also went on a date with one of the Mexican musicians from the house band. This young man took me to Puerto Marques for fresh clams on the half shell with limon and then took me to the Acapulco bullfights. Yikes! Well, that didn't work out so well, and afterwards I got very sick on our cab ride home. We pulled over so I could puke over the beautiful hillside above Puerto Marques. One day of bullfights was definitely enough for a lifetime.

It was a big treat for me when a friend of mine, Leopoldo "Polo" Farias III, from the USIU college system came to visit me from Mexico City, where he was living. He was just a good buddy from college. We were in different departments of the USIU school system, and he went to the business school on a soccer scholarship.

I hadn't seen him since I left school. He had decided to return to Mexico City with his family to finish his education. He was also a champion sailboat racer, and eventually a twelve times champion sailboat racer of Mexico. We went into town and had eats and Margaritas at Carlos and Charlies, where a year later my friends Sheryl and Alice Cooper (yes, THE Alice Cooper) would hold their wedding reception after their Acapulco wedding. Polo then went back to Mexico City. In another week, we'd be headed to Chicago.

I did almost make it thru Acapulco without Ray trying to worm his way into having sex with me, but a few weeks earlier, right before I got the crabs, he did call on the afternoon of a day off and ask if I would go to dinner with him.

"I've given you a good job with good money, don't you want to do something nice for me?" was his reasoning for the call. I took a deep breath and said, "Ray, do you recall what I told you when I accepted the offer to go on the road with you? DO YOU? Well, I meant it, so please no more calls unless it's something concerning the show. There are lots of other women out there (hookers, lol) who'd be thrilled to date you." And with that he said goodbye, and that was that forever. Yay! Chicago here we come.

What a shock to go to a climate as cold as Chicago after spending most of the winter in the tropics. Even though it was the first week in March, it was still freezing with some snow on the ground and the windchill coming off Lake Michigan was gruesome, probably about twenty degrees. We were booked into a somewhat rundown hotel, since the Playboy Club did not provide us with rooms, and Ray had to pay for them. We always had to buy our own food. My roommate was now Cozette, and we got along well.

We actually had a couple of days off before we restarted the show and the first thing I did was to go to Wilson's House of Suede and Leather, a famous chain store that sold mostly suede and leather coats, bags, hats etc., to look for a warm jacket. I found the cutest one I ever had, stylish beyond stylish. It was a waist-length jacket of patched colors of jewel tone leather sewn together randomly with white rabbit fur sleeves and a white rabbit fur bucket style hat to match, and it was warm. Nothing protects against wind chill like real fur. I this day and age, I hate to say it, but it's just the truth.

Then we went to the Playboy Building and Playboy Club to make sure we knew where we were working. Hugh Hefner grew up in Chicago and launched his magazine there. His first club was there, as was his first Playboy Mansion. The club was small and so was the stage and showroom compared to the Westside Room or the Acapulco Princess Showroom.

It was interesting working with the Bunnies and just sort of being in the ambiance of a gentleman's club, a different vibe. But it was all good and at least I was working. I had even paid off my college loan of $1,400 that I accrued from two years of private college. Amazing that it was so low, huh?

I turned 21 the week after we got to Chicago, and a bunch of us went to Benihana restaurant for my birthday, which began a lifelong love of Japanese cuisine. What delicious, healthy food, and I also learned to eat with chopsticks!

The Bunny "mother" was also nice, as were the Bunnies, who we became friendly with. The Bunny mother asked us if we wanted to come early one night before the show and be put in some Bunny costumes, and we all said YES! How fun. So, we did, and it was a trip: black sheer panty hose to the waist, then the satin bodysuit, high cut on the legs, and then stuffing the bras with clean remnants of black panty hose that had runs in them, cut up, to push up what tits you had. The reason black pantyhose was used to stuff our satin bras was that it cleverly didn't show at any angle in the low-cut top of the bodysuit.

After you were zipped in and pushed up, your tail was attached with two wide strips of Velcro. Lastly, the ears on a headband were placed on your head. Then came heels, and if you were a real Bunny, they had to be three inches and spotless. We took pictures and I didn't think any of us looked that great, as our legs were more muscular than the real Bunnies, and the suits just made them look huge. But we had a blast with that, and we were glad we did it.

Hugh Hefner never came to see our show, but ironically, I'd live at the Playboy Mansion West in L.A. six years later and become his brother Keith's girlfriend. But that's another story for later.

We finished our five-week run and then went on to Evansville, Indiana, for a week.

Evansville was our final booking on the tour and thank God for eight days only, as there was next to nothing to do there, at least that we had close access to. My Bookend friend, Carol Cali retaught me how to crochet, as my grandma Freida had taught me as a little girl, and the spring weather was nice to walk to work in.

Our venue was some sort of large Club that served alcohol, but the stage was rather small, and we could not do our kick ass Bobby Banas dance routines, just the previous dance routines and all our vocal numbers.

The owner of the Club had one of their female managers take the four of us Bookends out to a fine dining restaurant, and we all had lobster, which was the high point of my Evansville experience. Now, back to L.A.!

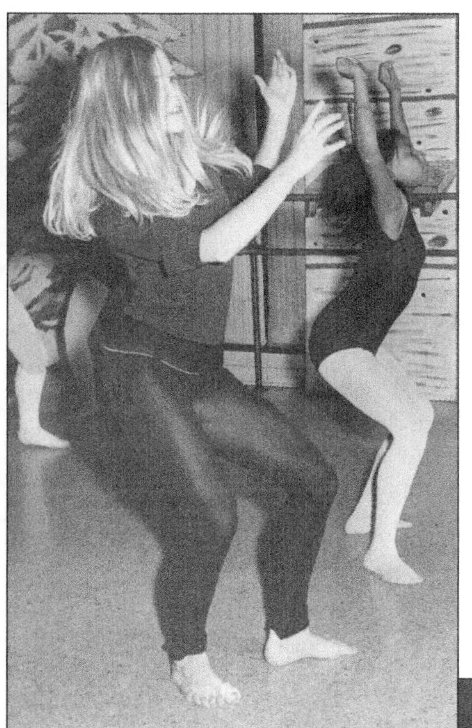

(Left) Jazz Dancing, Age 17,
In the Studio

(Below) My First Musical,
Guys and Dolls, Age 16,
West High School
with Bryan Solkowski

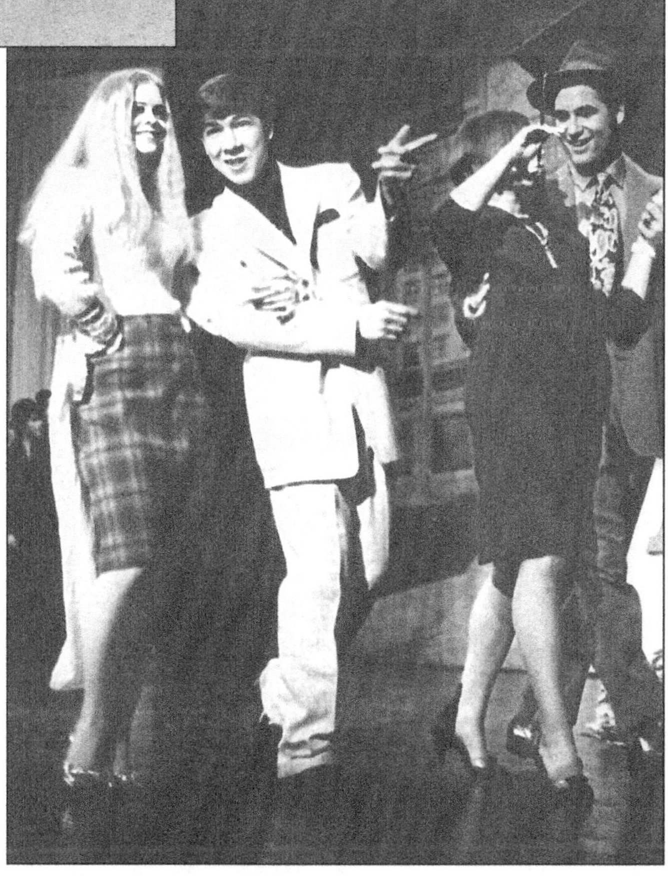

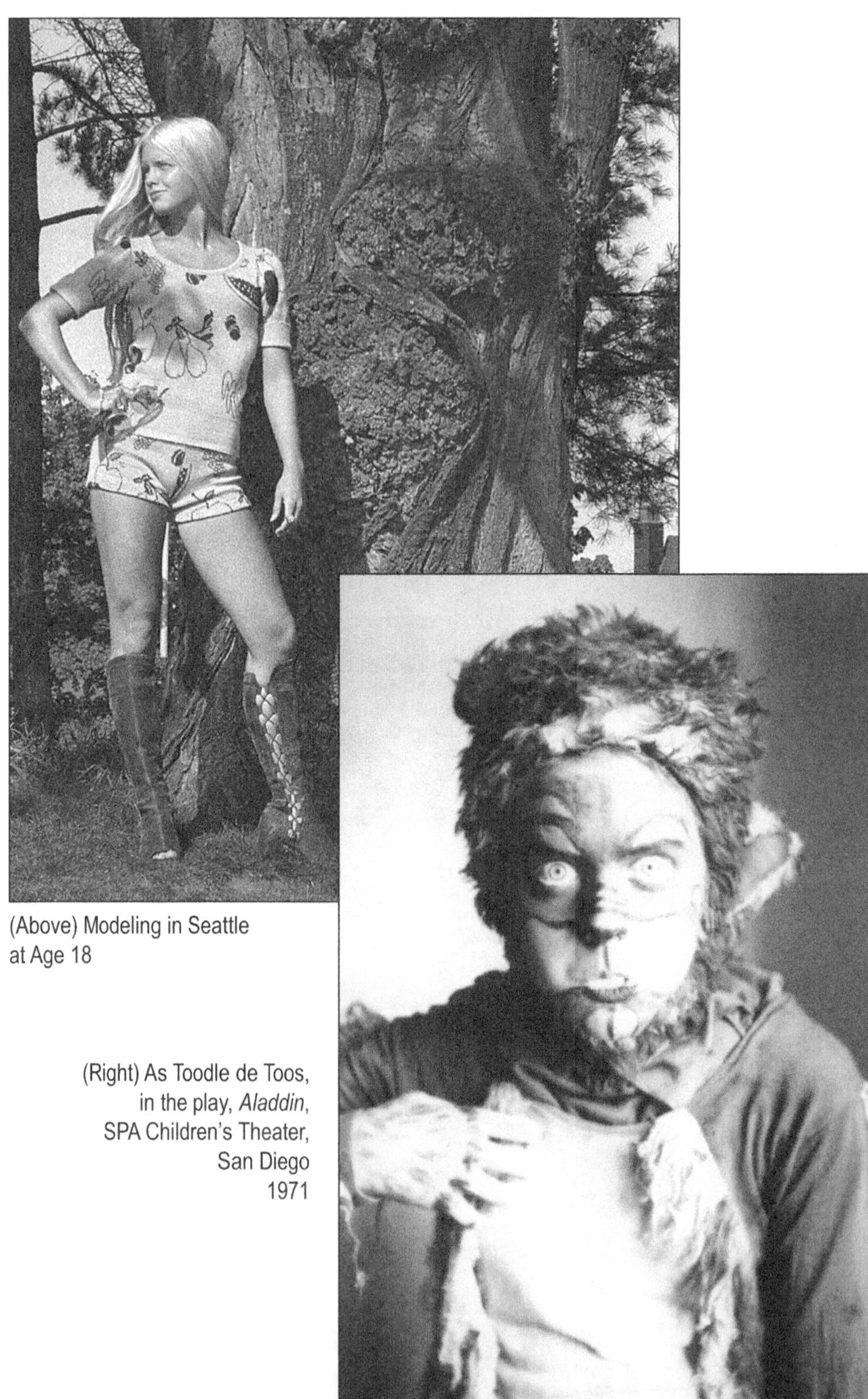

(Above) Modeling in Seattle
at Age 18

(Right) As Toodle de Toos,
in the play, *Aladdin*,
SPA Children's Theater,
San Diego
1971

All
of Us -
Dramatists
OC
1971
We
love
you!
4-Ever

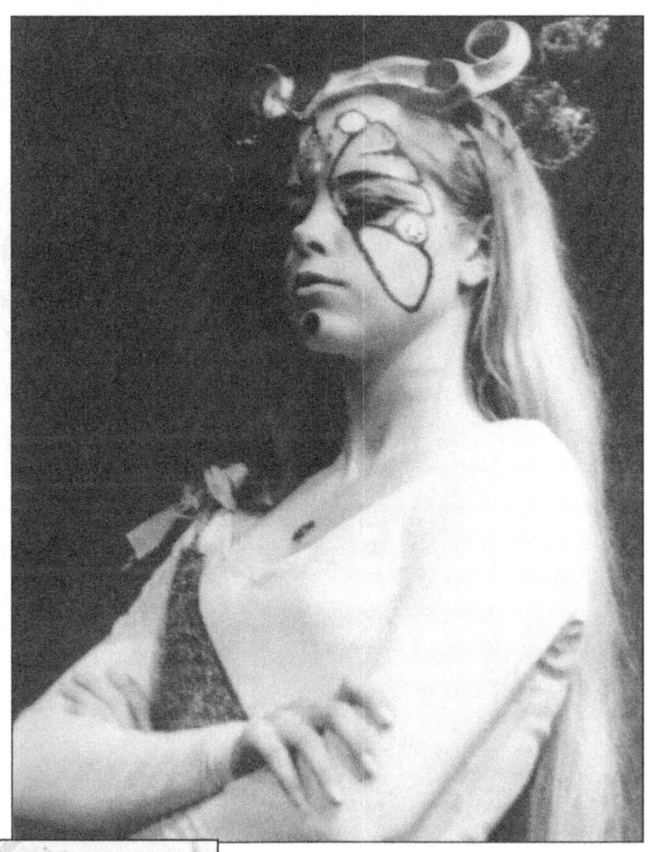

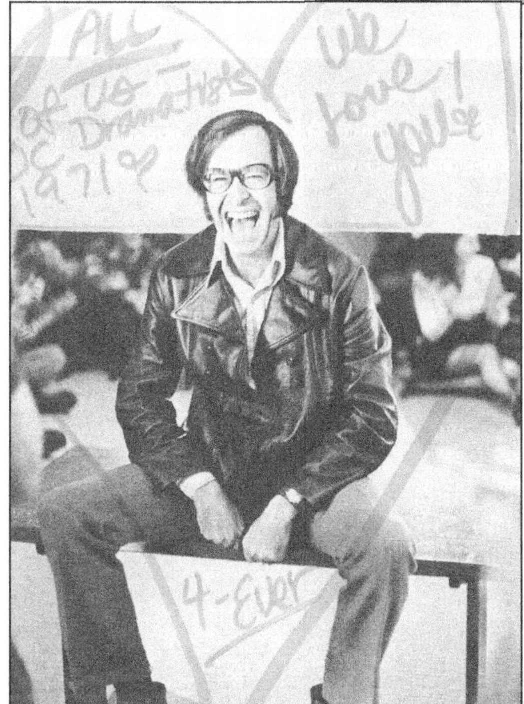

(Above) As Ariel in Shakespeare's
The Tempest,
Olympic College
1971

(Left) William "Bil" Harvey,
Acting Teacher and Director
at Olympic College
1971

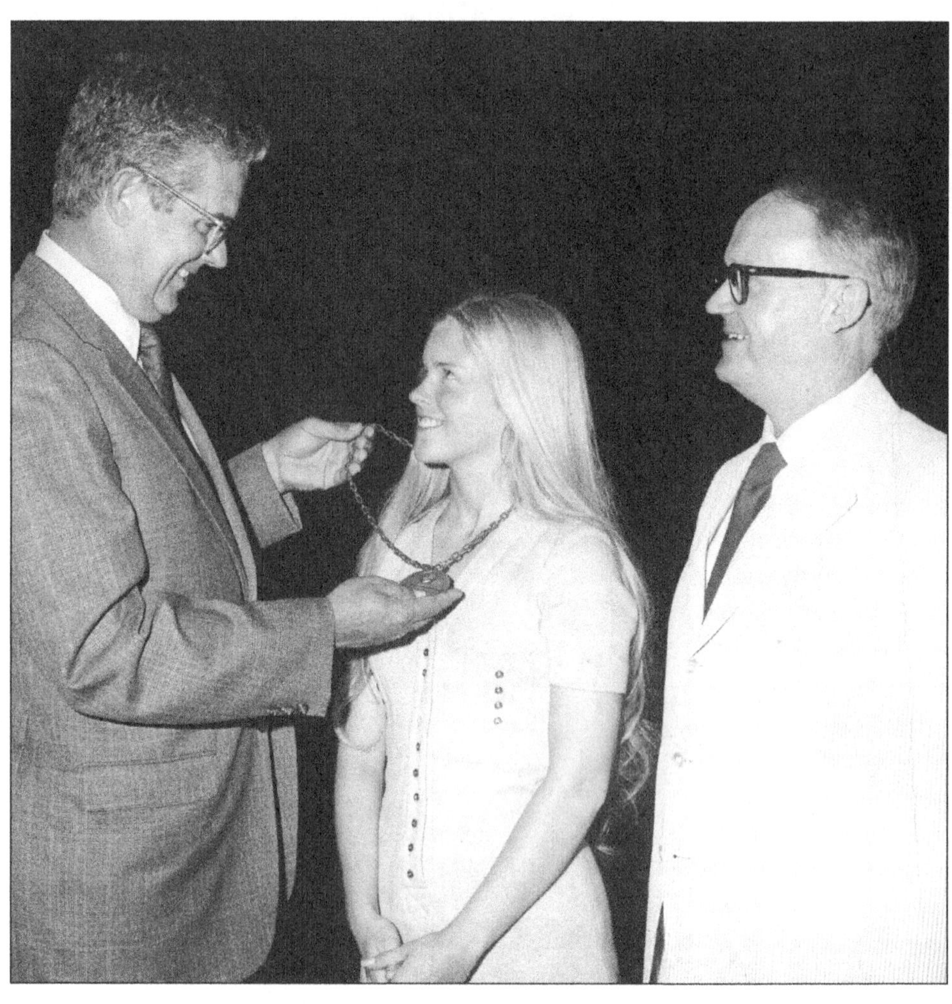

Receiving my Kennedy Center American College Theater Festival Award for *The Roar of the Greasepaint, The Smell of the Crowd*. 1972

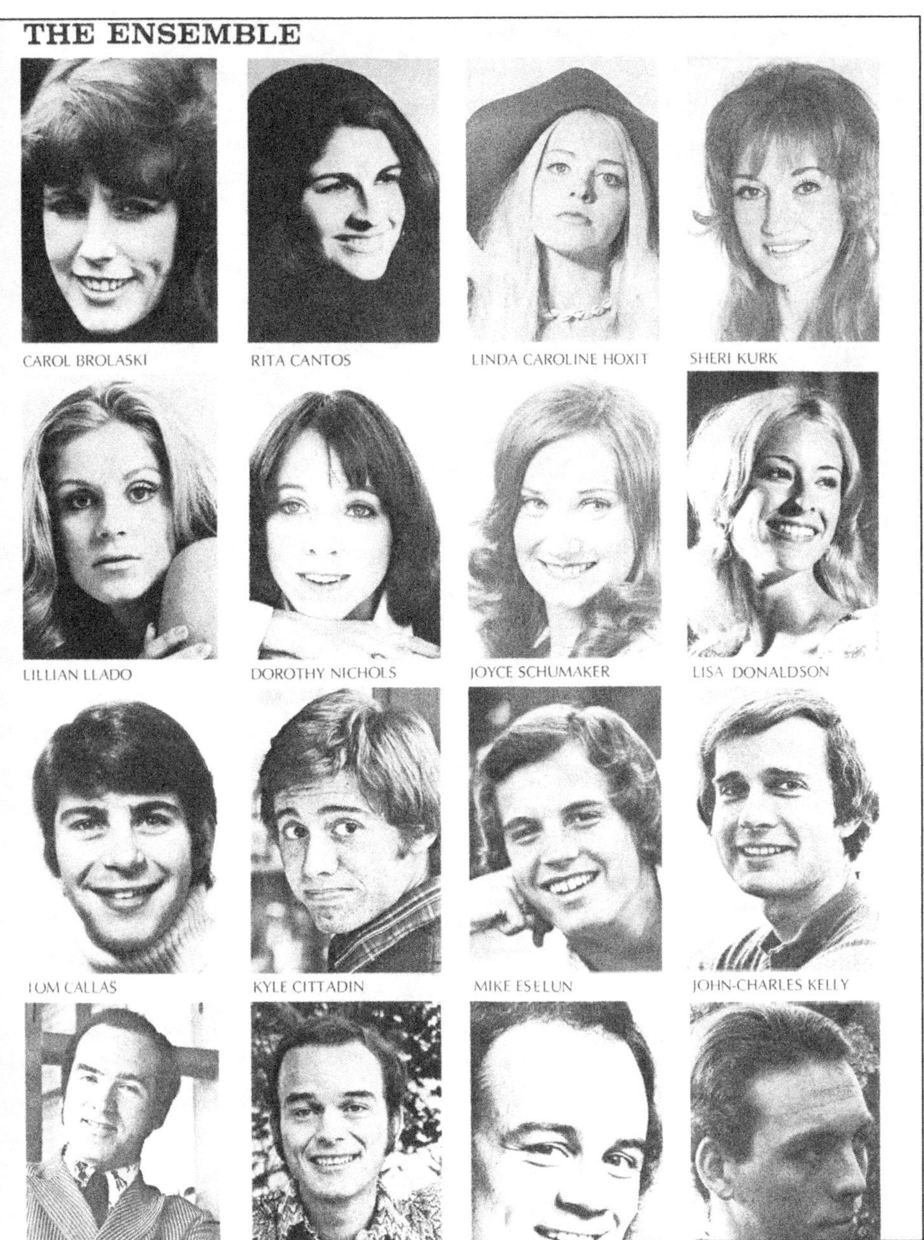

(Above) Sacramento Music Circus Ensemble Cast 1973

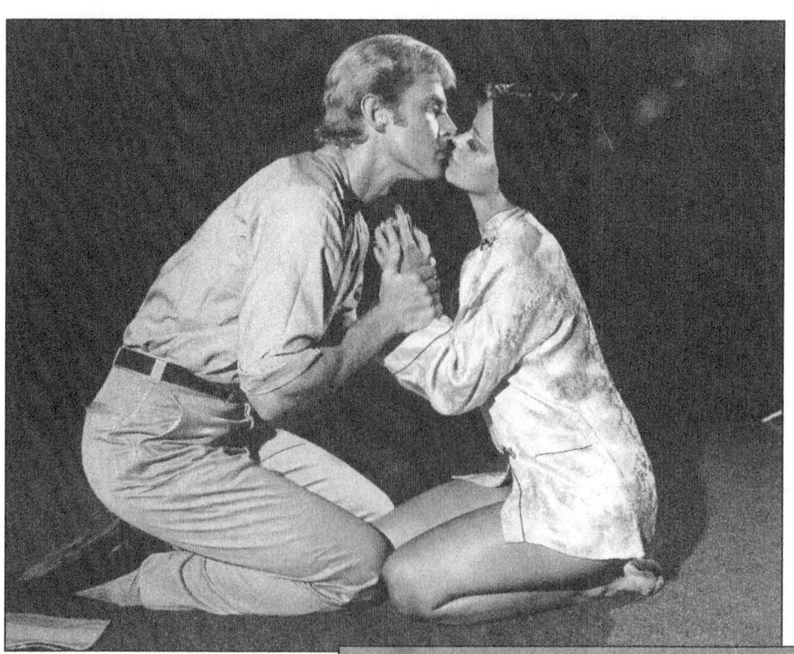

(Above) Brian Avery as Lt. Cable
and me as Liat, *South Pacific*,
Music Circus
1974

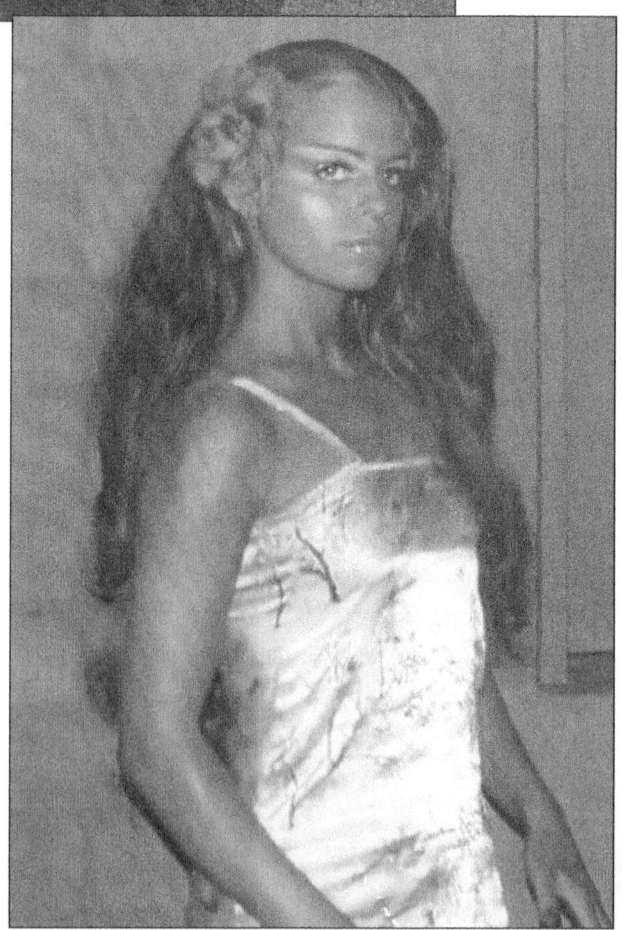

(Right)
As Liat, *South Pacific*,
Music Circus
1974

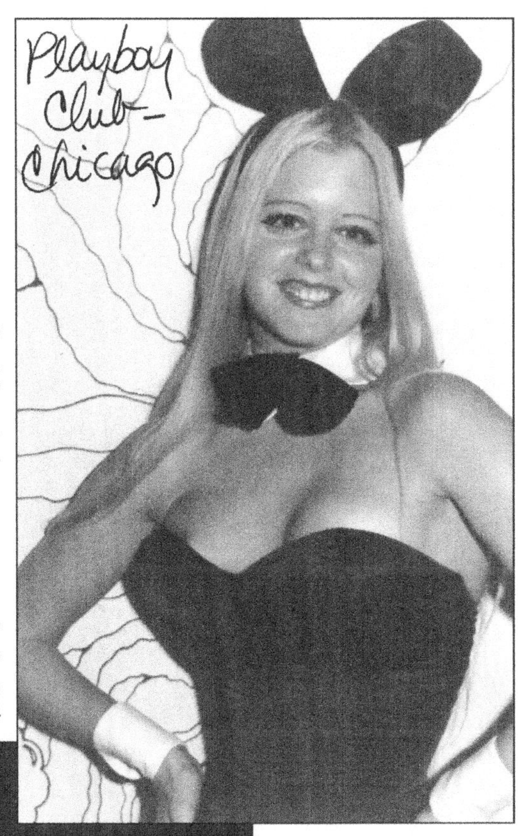

(Right) Working the Playboy Club in Chicago with the Bookends, dressed by the "Bunny Mother" in an authentic bunny costume. 1974

(Below) *The Student Prince*, as a German beerhall wench, Sacramento Music Circus, 1974

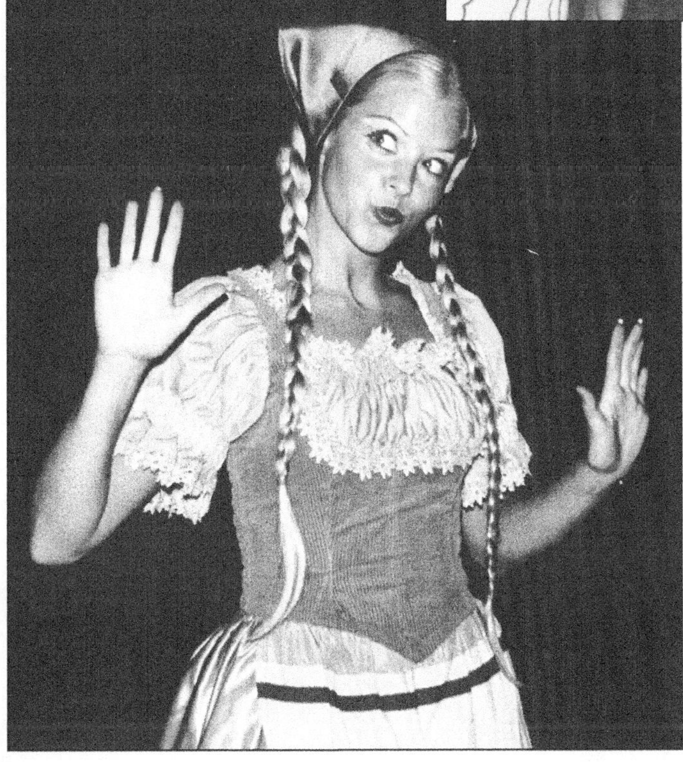

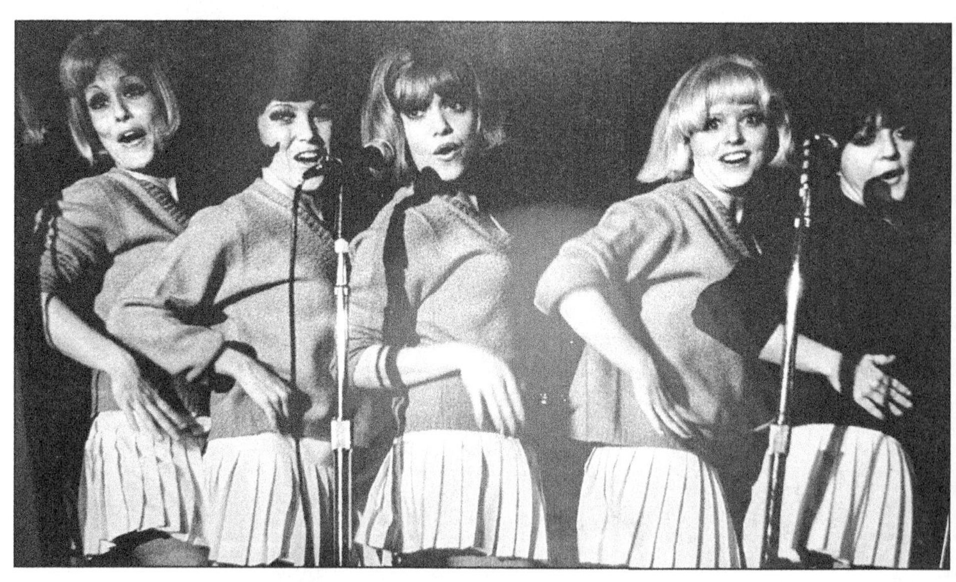

Ray Anthony's Bookends, "Jukebox Saturday Night" (I'm second from right.)

CHAPTER ELEVEN

I GET MY ROCK STAR

Back in L.A. and I'm staying with a quirky, funny girlfriend of mine, whose name escapes me, who was nice enough to keep my car in an underground parking garage. All my stuff was in the trunk of my Mustang except the clothes I took on the road.

She had a two-bedroom apartment in the well-known high rise apartment building located at the dead end of Fountain and Cahuenga. She's a secretary to a man who is a show biz manager, who wants to manage me, but I'm not really interested at this time, as I don't have much of a career to manage yet. I don't even have a single agent, let alone a manager!

It's the middle of April, and in June I will be going back to Sacramento to do another full season of Sacramento

Music Circus, offered to me at the end of the 1973 summer season. This time it's seven shows in eight weeks, three weeks longer than the '73 season.

After a couple of days reacclimating to L.A, doing laundry, buying groceries, I called Tony Lowe and Brantly Bright to see how they were doing. I had not communicated with them while on the road. Tony answered and he sounded sort of down, but happy to hear from me. He then informed me that Brantly had left L.A. to move back to Corpus Christi, her beautiful hometown, and her boyfriend from there, as well. L.A. just didn't hold that many opportunities for her, and she was homesick according to Tony. I understood that but felt bad for him—she was such a beauty!

He then asked me if I wanted to join him the following evening to go up and visit a friend of his in the Hollywood Hills. It was a musician/rock star named Al Kooper, who'd invited him up to hang at his house, have a drink, nothing special, just conversation.

Now I knew of Al Kooper from the late 60s. His album with the Blood, Sweat and Tears band had been quite popular, but I never bought it, although I liked it. So, I said sure. I just wanted to see Tony and be of some comfort to him. The next night, Tony picked me up. I dressed in the best casual pants outfit I had, plus my bunny fur leather coat.

We drove into the Hollywood Hills to a street off the famous Blue Jay Way of Beatles song fame. The house was very shlick with a pool out front. We were met by Al's bodyguard, Mickey Finn, a big burley man who was really a softie, but a bodyguard none the less. GEEZE!

He took us around the pool to a large sliding glass door and opened it to a sunken living room/dining room area. Up to the left was a higher platform area with a wall, floor to ceiling with record albums on shelves, and in front of that, with their backs towards us sitting at a white baby grand piano, was Al Kooper and a young blonde woman. He'd been playing something for her but stopped and turned to greet us as we came in.

Al looked just like he did on his album cover, *Child is Father to the Man*, with black curly hair but more like an afro now, as that photo was from '68, and it was now '74. He had an exotic look, with high cheekbones and deep-set eyes, not classically handsome, and he was rock star thin.

He and the blonde did not get up as Tony shook Al's hand and introduced me. I didn't shake his hand, not my style back then, and he looked happy to see me with a grin that showed sort of bad teeth. I smiled back and said, "Great to meet you," and meant it. He introduced Tony and me to the blonde gal as his date, and I forgot her name almost immediately, as I was in ecstasy, meeting my very first ROCK STAR!!!

Then Al rose and asked us if we wanted a glass of wine, but Tony would have to open the bottle, as Al did not drink ANYTHING except Keifer or water. When he was a young musician of 15, performing and touring with the band the Royal Teens, he drank hard alcohol and developed a chronic ulcer. This was rather refreshing for me—not the ulcer, but the fact he didn't drink.

So, Tony, the date, and I had a glass of white wine. We all moved down to the sunken part of the room that had a large semicircular couch. Tony and Al did most of the talking and the date and I were mostly quiet and listening. I found out Al had just turned 30 in February, and I'd just turned 21 in March.

Then somehow Al's date and Tony moved into the dining area to the left of the couch, and Al slid over on the couch closer to me. He started asking me questions and what I did for a living. "I'm one of Ray Anthony's Bookends at the moment, and I just got off the road with him and his band after four months," I informed him.

That really kicked it for Mr. Kooper, he could not believe it. "RAY ANTHONY? BIG BAND LEADER RAY ANTHONY???" I laughed and said, "Yup, we sing backup with him. We sing our own songs, and do dance routines, as well, but right now I'm on hiatus, and I'm going up to Sacramento the second week of June to do seven musicals with the Sacramento Music Circus summer stock company."

He quietly said, "Would you like to go to dinner with me tomorrow night and tell me more about yourself? I'm a member of a private exclusive dinner club called PIPS in Beverly Hills. I can take you. You'll like it, but you'll have to drive up here and we'll take the Silver Cloud to the club."

Alrighty then, woo hoo! He wrote down his phone number on a piece of paper and said, "Call me midday tomorrow and we'll set a time, and I'll give you directions on how to get up here."

Then we went down to Tony and Al's date, and I had a cigarette and we all just continued to make small talk, while I tried not to look like a smitten teenager. After about a half hour, Tony announced he had an early photo shoot in the morning (Emerson-Lowe Photography, specializing in the music industry), and needed to get some shuteye, so we split. On the ride home, I told Tony what had transpired between Al and me, and he admitted that HE was attracted to Al's blonde date and got her information. Well good for US!

I called Al, got the directions, and drove up the Hollywood Hills to his house the next evening. There was an open carport with Al's two cars to the right, and a truck to the left which Al had told me to park behind.

The bodyguard, Mickey (Frank Sinatra's prior bodyguard), came out to escort me in, and Al came out of his bedroom on the far left. He had a denim jacket on, with all sorts of various wild bird feathers attached to the lapel and some groovy looking leather pants, vavavoom! We said goodbye to Mickey, and went to Al's Silver Cloud Rolls Royce, which was parked behind the Citroen Maserati. Of course, I sat right next to my date, as was the custom of that time.

We got down to the club in the middle of Beverly Hills. I loved the look of it. It was all dark wood, with low lighting. He ordered the lamb chops and recommended I do the same. I had a glass of wine, and he had milk. Throughout my dance career, I cut way back on red meat, maybe once a month, and so it was extra delicious.

When we finished dinner, we went back up to Al's house and then he said he wanted to play piano for me. We sat on the bench together just like he had with his date the night before. After a few minutes, he suggested we move down to the sunken part of the living room on the couch and let the making out begin.

The chemistry was electric. As the situation started to heat up, I pulled back and stopped the progress of what was sure to be lovemaking. "I'm going to need to go home soon, I don't go all the way on a first date." That was my rule back then and I didn't have my protection in, as well. "I really like you and I'm very attracted to you but just not tonight."

He wasn't mad. "Okay, okay," he said, "but how about dinner again in two nights? I have a recording session tomorrow night. We'll have dinner in and you will spend the night, won't you?"

I laughed a hearty laugh and said, "Absolutely, I'll be counting the minutes."

I got in my car and went home reluctantly, as I did want Rock Star sex something awful!

Two days have gone by, and it's Friday night. I make sure to have my flying saucer baby stopper ready to go and my prettiest lingerie on, and Mickey lets me in per usual. I finally meet the live-in maid, a young black woman who is talkative and very nice. The maid and butlers' quarters are down at the other end of the house, just past a game room, complete with pool table and a pinball machine.

She had set the dining room table and there were Chinese takeout boxes unopened and a bottle of wine in a bucket with ice, which she said Mickey had opened for me. On the table there were candles burning, although it was still daylight out.

Al comes out of the bedroom dressed casually in a pair of jeans and an open chiffon-style shirt that showed his very flat stomach and thin physique. I had never really been attracted to meaty, muscular men. I liked the thin artistic-style bodies, at least 5'10" to no more than about 6'1", dark hair, and large eyes. He was perfect.

The maid left us alone and we ate, and I hardly remember what the food even tasted like. After eating, we didn't even go to the couch, just straight for the bedroom.

It had a huge king-size bed and an attached master bathroom with a sunken tub. We practically ripped our clothes off and jumped under the sheets to do some passionate necking and petting and then I went down on him and his well-endowed person. I was decent at head, and he seemed to enjoy it, and then I was on top of him with him in me which was a relatively new position for me, but definitely pleasurable and erotic.

We stopped for a few minutes to prolong the experience, and I was supporting myself with my hands on his shoulders looking at his fabulous face and he said, "Lin, I LOVE YOU, Lin." I audibly gasped. I was speechless and gave him a prolonged French kiss instead. No boyfriend had EVER told me they loved me.

We finished our lovemaking, fairly exhausted, and we rested for a bit before we went again, until sleep came and stole us away for the night in each other's arms. I had found heaven on earth, and I even liked the way he smelled. When we awoke and made love again, he asked me if I'd like to move in with him. I had not even known him for a week, but I really didn't have much to lose. I was still at my friend's apartment, and my only other option was getting a place of my own, so I said, "Okay, let's give it a go!" The worst that could happen was I'd just get a place of my own if it didn't work out, right?

I had breakfast and took a bath in the sunken tub. After leaving, I went to Ralphs supermarket and bought some flowers for my friend for allowing me to crash with her. I packed the rest of my stuff in my Mustang and headed on up to Al's to begin my four-and-a-half-year journey with him. I got my Rock Star.

CHAPTER TWELVE

LIFE WITH ALLIE AND LYNYRD SKYNYRD

So, I drag my clothes into our bedroom and leave the rest of my stuff in the car trunk for now. There was another car in the driveway that somehow escaped my attention, a sort of beat up 1972 Corvette, metallic blue. Anyway, I'm slowly learning what goes on here as I unpack my wardrobe. The maid helps everyone with breakfast and will also help with lunch if you want it.

She and Mickey disappear to their part of the house by about 5pm, where they have a small kitchen and bedrooms with baths attached, with the game room between them and us. Al filled me in on Mickey and the maid's relationship, as they fought verbally frequently, which I soon experienced. She was very talkative, and it irritated Mickey.

Al and I have a "food discussion" and I find out he prefers to do most of his own cooking with his chronic ulcer and said I should also get some food for myself. I found a Gelson's nearby in Hollywood, and bought some salmon, yogurt, coffee, and salad ingredients, just enough for a few days. Mickey helped me in with my grocery bags. Al was in the kitchen making homemade chicken soup, one of his staples, and Al offered me some of his soup and it was very tasty. He told me he'd teach me how to make it, and he eventually did.

Then it was time for "snoogling" (cuddling) on the couch, but nothing sexual, just hugging which we both LOVED. I had bought a salmon fillet and potatoes, so I fixed that, and Al could eat that. He then told me about his latest project, producing a band from the Southern United States with an odd name called Lynyrd Skynyrd. He showed me the two albums he'd produced for them and played some of their songs for me. The music was fairly foreign to me. I just nodded my head and smiled and didn't say much, as I was very into the British Invasion at that time, like the Stones and Rod Stewart.

We retired early and had more passionate sex, and this was our routine for the next couple of days. We were eating dinner on the third night, and he looked me in the eyes and said he had to tell me something that I really needed to know. "I love you, I do, it was love at first sight for me but ..." He paused, then continued. "I have an impossible time being faithful to my women. After two marriages and two divorces, it is an incurable character trait of mine. I'm not going to lie, and it won't be often, and I will not have an affair, only one-time flings. There are women called groupies, and sometimes I can't resist."

He stopped and waited for a response from me. I needed a moment or three to process this, but I did appreciate his courage and transparency. In my head, I thought, "He'll grow out of this, I will love it out of him and he's young yet, he'll get tired of these floozies with so little self-respect." That was my inner dialogue.

My only other option was to say, "No thanks, not interested," and once again, rent a place of my own, or ride it out, and see what eventually transpired. The fact that I would be leaving for Sacramento and living there for two full months was sort of like that anyway.

I finally opened my mouth and my response was this: "I'm so madly in love with you I can hardly see straight, and I believe this will work for now as long as what you say about not having an affair is true." And Al responded, "I swear it, it will be so brief and so few you won't even know it happened, and I won't tell you as it will mean nothing to me but a sexual encounter."

Now this was the 70s when there was a definite sexual progressiveness and open mindedness the world had never really experienced before—group sex, open marriages, wife swapping and the like, none of which interested me at all. But I was NOT leaving him, "wild horses" and all that.

I needed to go to Moro Landis dance studio and take some classes, mainly jazz dance from Bobby Banas, or my new fave, Joe Tremaine. I wasn't currently auditioning for anything, as I was contracted with Music Circus for another full summer of seven musicals.

Al told me Lynyrd Skynyrd was coming to town and was playing at the Santa Monica Civic Auditorium. He said we'd be going to and see them, but first they were coming up to the house in the next couple of days to sign a contract for their third album with him.

Sure enough, a Lincoln town car came up to the house, dumping out six of the most long-haired young men I'd ever seen, with hair down past their shoulders, and acting rather wildly. The lead singer grabbed my hand and kissed it and said, "Pleased to meet you, ma'am," and if my pants hadn't been buttoned, they'd have fallen to my knees. How fucking charming was that??? Al said jokingly "You've got to watch this one." Although he wasn't very good looking and was slightly chubby, Ronnie Van Zant had a certain savoir faire and self confidence that made him feel like a Rock Star.

Al and I dressed in our hippie finest, and took a limo, yes, a black limousine to the Civic. We had no seats, just backstage passes that we attached to our clothes where they could be seen. We went directly to a lounge close to the stage. It had couches and chairs, and a large case of Jack Daniels and glasses, with ice and bottles of water, nothing else. There with their guitars were Ronnie, Allen, Billy, Ed, Robert, Gary and Leon (Gary and Leon were the most attractive). Of course, Ronnie stood up when I entered the room and came over and took my hand and kissed it and said "ma'am." It was about forty-five minutes until showtime, so we sat down with them.

I was offered a glass of JD, and I joined them in their pre-show drinking and smoking cigarettes. A few of them had their own bottles and were drinking straight from them. I needed some ice with mine. I'd never had whiskey before, YOWZA!

I gingerly sipped my drink, but they just slugged it down. I'm glad I did though, because what was to come was a bit hard for even a concert veteran like me to take. So, the stage manager came back and told them it was time to start, and we went with them to the side of the stage. The emcee introduced them, and the capacity crowd went nuts as they ran out onstage, while Al and I stayed standing on the side.

They ripped into "Workin' for MCA," which was their usual opening song, and MY GOD, they were soooo loud. I wasn't familiar with their music at all, but one song was catchy, called "Sweet Home Alabama." Their finale, "Freebird," was long and dynamic.

The long-legged lead guitar player, Allen, with his long, long hair flying, did a large vertical leap in the air, at a dramatic chord close to the end of the long instrumental portion of the eleven-minute song. Then at the end, all four guitar players were downstage, playing the hard rock intensely and swaying front and back in unison, with a dramatic drum and guitar ending.

The set was an hour and forty-five minutes, and my ears were just ringing and would continue to ring for the next few hours. It was shell shock for me, but they were good musicians and Ronnie was a sexy, suave Southern front man with his signature black hat and bare feet, with jeans and a worn tee shirt. I knew they'd become big stars and of course they did.

We said our goodbyes and Al said, "See you in three weeks." We were going to see them in Atlanta at one of their first stadium shows as headliners.

I'd been with Al about a month now, and this was our first actual trip together. We flew first class on Delta to Atlanta, complete with steak dinners, all the champagne one could drink, and topped off with an ice cream sundae cart! A limo picked us up and took us to the Hyatt Regency, with its signature garden interior and visible elevators in glass tubes. The entire band was staying there too.

We arrived a day ahead of them, and the band manager had an open house in his room, for just hanging out and schmoozing, which Al did more than me. I didn't mind. I went walking around outside to get a sense of this beautiful Southern city, as I'd never been to the Southern U.S. before.

The next day, around noon, we all got in limos with the band and headed to Fulton County Stadium. It was June 1st, 1974. It was a daytime concert that started at around 4pm, and the band needed to do a sound check. The stadium held around fifty to sixty thousand people and was just massive. The backstage area had dressing rooms and a full lounge/cafeteria area with a delicious buffet and all sorts of beverages, not just Jack Daniels this time. We sure partook of that!

The Charlie Daniels Band was the opening act. They went on first at about 3:15 and played for about thirty minutes. They were a hit with the massive audience, Skynyrd, and Al.

The equipment change took about fifteen minutes, and a large confederate flag went up behind Robert's drum kit, flying in the breeze, a good backdrop, I had to admit.

Then they were announced, and a roar went up, much like when I saw the Beatles in Seattle, and I realized just how popular they had become. It was a totally open-air stadium so this was to be much more enjoyable than the Santa Monica Civic. The searing electric guitar music had somewhere to go.

Some of the audience left their seats and formed a large mosh pit in front of the stage. Being so close must have been more fun for the big, drunk or stoned group of young Skynyrd fans. This time I really enjoyed them, and I was getting familiar with their music. They moved around well and presented themselves with a lot of confidence. They were really entertaining to watch. They played for about an hour and a half, ending with "Freebird," which I was totally into now, with Allen Collins' big jump, guitar in hand and hair flying, and the four guitars down stage at the end, just shredding their parts.

We all went back to the Hyatt where there was more food and beverages set up in a large room, along with the smoking of weed and more Jack Daniels, just not for me. Some of their wives and girlfriends had come to join them from Jacksonville, Florida, their hometown, but they did not have their three background singers yet, the Honketts. They would be added in another couple of months.

It was such a heady experience to see this band rising to fame and fortune, and so well deserved. They were so tight, so talented, and there was no other music quite like theirs, except The Allman Brothers Band. Al and I said our fond farewells and flew Delta back to L.A. the next day, and the band headed out for more dates on the road.

CHAPTER THIRTEEN

THE SCARIEST NIGHT OF MY LIFE

I was starting to have all sorts of car problems with my 1965 Mustang convertible. It was nine years old, and even though I'd had the oil changes with regularity, it was failing.

So, Al asks me if I'd like to have the Corvette! Well, once again, I didn't have a lot of money for a new car, so sure, why not? He had driven it out from Atlanta when he was living there for two years, just before he moved to L.A., and he admittedly didn't take very good care of it.

I drove it down to a service station in Hollywood and had the oil changed. but the engine still ran rough. The service station owner, who had been friendly to me and recognized me, asked about my Mustang, and said, "What up with the Corvette?"

I told him, and he said he wanted to buy the Mustang from me. He offered me $150 for it, so I said fine. I'd only paid $700 for it anyway, so done deal. I was going to have a long drive up to Sacramento in about two weeks for the summer, as well. I went home and transferred my meager amount of household goods in the trunk to the trunk of the Corvette, took it to the service station, collected my money, and he drove me home.

On that Friday, after we got home, Al got a call from Gary Kellerman, the very sleazy half owner of the very outrageous recording studio for rockers, The Record Plant. The Record Plant was a state-of-the-art recording studio with the best sound equipment and latest technology. It also had offices for deal making, hanging out, a jacuzzi, and two bedrooms for naps if needed. But really, it was more for sexual encounters with groupies. One was an S&M-style bedroom with whips and such on the walls that I found out later was nicknamed "The Al Kooper Memorial Bedroom." Jesus!

Gary was the wild, drug-ridden owner of the Record Plant and his partner Chris Stone was the responsible businessman and family man. Gary told Al that Ronnie Wood of the Stones (newly inducted and lured away from Faces) and Rod Stewart and his wife Chrissie were in town and there was a party at Alice Cooper's house somewhere in the Canyons. He said to come down about 6:00 to the studio, pick them up, and come with them.

Sure 'nuf, we put on some wild clothes and got in the Silver Cloud and headed on down to the studio on 3rd Street in the Melrose District. The three of them got in the back seat, and I was thrilled to meet Ron Wood. I'd been around him once in Seattle, a couple of years earlier. After the Rod Stewart/Faces concert in Seattle, there was a party at The Edgewater Inn, where I saw him briefly. It was down by the Bremerton Ferry we were taking back home.

I wasn't going to bring that up and sound like a groupie, especially in front of his delicate, beautiful blonde British wife. Ronnie was always cute at that time, with jet black hair in the fashionable pineapple haircut, like Rod Stewart. He was always smiling, happy, and congenial for being so famous.

Gary then told Al and me that Ronnie and Chrissie had a big bag of cocaine in her purse that we could all imbibe when we got to Alice's party. I'd experimented with drugs in high school, but I'd never even had a line of blow. So, we're on Sunset, getting ready to go up Laurel Canyon, when a cop car suddenly pulls up behind us with flashing lights, for us to pull over.

Oh no, oh no, oh no, no, no, no, no! Al was very polite, and said, "Hi Officer, what's wrong?" smiling at him. "You changed lanes and didn't put on your turn signal. License and registration please," was the officer's reply.

Al gave them to him, and the cop went to his car to see if there were any outstanding warrants on Al, and we were all collectively holding our breath, eyes big as dinner plates. If he searches us and finds the coke, we ALL go to jail, as it's an illegal schedule two narcotic.

So, the cop returns and gives Al his documents back and says, "Okay, just a warning this time, but next time be more aware of that," and he shined his flashlight in and looked at all of us, as it was dusk.

We were all very quiet and politely smiling. We couldn't have looked more liberal and rocker if we tried. At least no one had whipped out a joint for him to smell. We dodged a bullet on that. We waited for him to leave, and we all started breathing again and commented on Al's cool behavior, and we were all so grateful and relieved.

We turned right and found the street off Laurel Canyon and the address Gary had. We found the house with a lot of cars parked in front, and went in. It was odd-ish, with loud music playing, and a lot of, sort of crazed-looking people drinking and smoking weed, etc.

Some guy who seemed to be in charge greeted us. Gary asked, "Where's Alice?" and he said, "Oh, he's in Vegas working, but this is his rental, and he just told us to have a good time." HMMMM? The house was very spartan, with no artwork on the walls, just some tables and chairs and stereo equipment. But Al, Ronnie, Chrissie, and I didn't like the vibe. It just felt wrong to be in somebody's house when they weren't there, especially with narcotics. We told Gary and said we could go back up to our house and they could come with, but Gary wanted to stay. Ronnie and his wife would join us.

We drove back to our house in the Hollywood Hills. Ronnie asked if he could open the baggie of coke, and Al took him to the kitchen where Ron dumped the entire large baggie on the cutting board on the island in the kitchen.

The dollar bills came out and I watched Ron and wife imbibe. The dollar bills were then passed to Al and me and Al politely said no because of his ulcer. I looked at Al and said something like "Is this, okay?" and he said, "Go for it," so, yup I did.

We had some wine, smoked a lot of cigarettes, (Al did join us for that), listened to music from the large wall of records, and had a great time. Around 3am, everybody started to poop out, so we got a cab for Ronnie and Chrissie to go back to their hotel, and that was that. I never saw either of them again, but I will always remember that night, and how lucky we were!

I have about four days until I leave for Sacramento Music Circus. I was sad about leaving Al, but our love was strong, and I knew we'd be okay. I needed to work. I did not just want to be a man's stay-at-home wife, as I'd worked so hard to get into show biz. I was looking forward to seeing my cast from last summer, and Jack Bunch, our wonderful director, and choreographer Walter Painter, and Lewis & Young.

The Friday before I was heading up, driving the Corvette this time, I'd packed most of my clothes and put them in the trunk with my survival housewares. I had secured a studio apartment in the same complex that I had last year, with just the same meager furniture and murphy bed.

That morning, Al told me that a photographer named Norman Seeff would be up to the house that afternoon to do a photo shoot with Al. Norman was a rock photographer from South Africa, who had done album covers for Skynyrd and many other bands and solo artists. He was putting together a book of famous clients called *Hot Shots* that would include Al, as well.

It was a gorgeous late spring day, and I just wanted to hang by the pool. I had packed my one bikini in a suitcase, and didn't want to get it out, lazy me, so I was sunbathing in a pair of black underwear and a white bra.

Norman shows up about three and he's an interesting man. I continued to sunbathe for another quarter of an hour or so, and then I came into the living area to watch. Norman had set up some lights facing the wall of records behind it. It was good for a backdrop. Al had also been sunbathing that morning and had shorts on and a bare chest with a tanned body and his big poufy afro that I loved.

Al offered Norman a drink and he said, "I'll have a whiskey if your girlfriend here will join me," so I said okay, thinking, "Oh shit," but at least I had it on the rocks.

Norman takes some shots of Al in the big armchair, but it was sort of boring, I had to admit. I was starting to feel warm from the drink and Norman suggested I come over and sit by Al in the armchair. I put the drink down and joined Al. The shot of us that Norman chose for the book was perfect! I looked coy and my legs were covering my body, with Al, sort of turned away from me, with a very mischievous look on his face.

Norman took a few more of both of us, and then Al had his first ulcer attack since we were together and excused himself to go to the bathroom for a while. So, I was there with Norman and our drinks, and we started talking. He asked what my trip was, and I said, "Mostly a dancer, and I do musicals, dancing & singing." Then he said, "Let's do a couple of dance shots of you in the chair while we wait for Al to feel better." By then I was tipsy and feeling no pain, so I got wild and crazy on the chair, and encouraged by Norman to make a crazy face, I did, tongue waaaay out!

Al really did not feel well and bowed out of the rest of the session but came back out to say goodbye as Norman packed up his gear and split.

His photo book came out and it was a big hit. I wasn't the only one in underwear, Carly Simon was too. John Mayall was completely nude in a swimming pool, being held up by girls. Davey Jones, with the other Monkees, hung a bare assed moon, and there were many other amusing shots of rock stars and sometimes their women, in humorous or candid poses. Norman's style was known as "mucous focus," as he used a lot of diffusion and all black and white at that time. Our pages are 38 and 39, with me getting an extra page. In 1974, it was the first book I was ever in, and the most embarrassing photo of my life.

CHAPTER FOURTEEN

MUSIC CIRCUS, SUMMER OF 1974

I hug and kiss the love of my young life goodbye, and he promises he'll come and visit me in a few weeks. He warns me he does NOT like musicals, and I tell him I don't that much either, but it's what I am trained to do, so I'm not going to waste my education.

I get into my metallic blue Chevrolet Corvette and head north to Sacramento. At least it has air conditioning, as my Mustang did not. The seven-hour drive is not all that bad, and I stop for lunch and gas up halfway. It amazes me to this day that I had no fear of that. The freeways were not as crazy and crowded back then like they are today, and I would go long stretches where I'd virtually be alone for miles and miles.

I got to my old apartment on G Street, and the apartment manager showed me to this year's apartment, which is on the second floor. (Last year, I was on the first floor.) I dragged my stuff up the stairs and prepared my murphy bed and took a nap. After that, I went to the store, bought food, collapsed and slept some more. I will also get a phone this year, so I can call Al from time to time. You had to pay extra for long distance back then, plus I would be working day and night.

I got up early for the first time in about two months, made coffee and a muffin, put my dance clothes on, and walked the two blocks to the tent. I was delighted to see so many smiling, familiar faces, but realized that about half the chorus from last year did not accept the offer to return without having to audition again, which I thought was a shame since they were all so fun, so nice.

One of the new chorus members was Carol Lugenbeal, "Luge" as we called her at SPA, and I was happy to see her. So, I had one other SPA alum to work with. Dorothy Nichols, Chuck Spoerri, Sheri Kirk, and Kyle Cittadin returned also, but the other eleven did not. It was sort of shocking, and who knew why? All of the new eleven were talented and congenial, as were choreographer, Walter Painter and director, Jack Bunch.

Our first show of the summer was *Once Upon a Mattress* starring the hilarious Jo Ann Worley, and Henry Gibson as the Prince to her Winifred. It was a fun, silly show, and I loved singing "I'm in Love with a Girl named Fred, with an F and an R and an E and a D, and a F R E D, FRED." Always a party with Jo Ann!

Our second musical was *Gigi* starring Howard Keel, Terrence Monk, and Loni Ackerman as Gigi. An interesting thing happened: Walter got a job offer to choreograph Ann- Margret's act in Vegas, as he had been one of her backup dancer boys, leaving Lewis & Young high and dry with next to no notice. He was scheduled to work the entire summer, which I thought was pretty shitty of him, but hell, what did I know? Didn't he have a contract? The rest of us did.

His replacement, Carl Jablonski, who none of us knew, was from L. A. and had done mostly TV choreography. He did not choose us and sometimes directors and choreographers have a hard time with that as they may not click with the talent, and I think he did have a hard time.

We dancer girls started off by rehearsing the opening can-can dance for the very Parisian show, and he asked us if we could all do running front handsprings, and we could! Except they were down one of the main aisles to the stage at about a 25-degree angle, and no exact counts, just the three main dancers going one after another.

Well, you're not supposed to run a horse downhill, and you shouldn't do gymnastics close together or downhill, but we just did as we were told. I was behind Dorothy, and hit her on the head with my foot, in my character heels. The rehearsal was called to a halt, and Dorothy had to sit down, now crying. I hurt her and felt like shit!

That was quickly changed to running down to the stage doing the can-can skirt thing—left and right—but I wondered why this man had tried to do the handsprings at all, as there is that thing called gravitational pull, and it was just not safe. We did a second can-can that was challenging and fun.

The stars were all very talented. One of the other cast members had told me Terrence Monk, who was playing Gaston, had a crush on me. Sure enough, I saw him watching me and our eyes met, and we both smiled. He was a handsome man in his 30s, but of course I was with Al, so nothing happened with us.

Interestingly, my future second husband, Alan Almeida, at the age of 17 had been cast in a bit role in *Gigi*, with his claim to fame, serving a salad to Howard Keel, who was playing Honoré. Soon after, he was hired as a production assistant by day, and a stagehand by night for the remainder of the season. Years later, when we connected, he showed me my autograph in his program, so we did encounter each other, but never actually met at the time. He admitted having a boyhood crush on me back then, too.

Musical number three was *On a Clear Day You Can See* Forever, which starred Lainie Kazan and Jerry Lanning. We marveled at how "voluptuous" Lainie Kazan was in her tight jeans—to be polite. She did have a wonderful voice. The chorus had next to nothing to do. We did one dance step across the stage. Anyway, we did a lot of clowning around backstage on this show as we had so little to do, the part of theater that I loved—screwing around backstage.

Musical number four was *My Fair Lady*. Our stars were Michael Allinson as Henry Higgins, Karen Morrow, as Eliza Doolittle, and a handsome blonde singer/actor, Brian Avery, as Freddy Eynsford-Hill. They were all very good in their respective roles.

Most musicals are either dancing musicals or singing musicals, very few are equal parts singing AND dancing. *My Fair Lady* was most definitely a singing musical and we had such a good time singing "Ascot Gavotte." We were in really heavy 19th century costumes up to our necks, with huge hats and parasols in the Sacramento heat!

Since there was so little dancing, we hardly interacted with Carl Jablonski, but then he had to leave for a previous obligation back in L.A., and we were left without a choreographer again.

Musical number five was *South Pacific*. At the end of *On a Clear Day*, right before we started rehearsals for *South Pacific* and opened *My Fair Lady*, I was asked to go and talk to Howard and Russell in their office—mysterious, but nothing negative, a good vibe. I sat down opposite them at their desks and Russell said, "We made a hiring error and forgot to hire a Liat for *South Pacific*. We think you could play her. Would you be interested to do so?"

I smiled and said, "Who is Liat? I've never seen *South Pacific*." "She's the Polynesian ingenue who falls in love with the young lieutenant male principal in the story, and she dances," replied Howard.

"I'm hardly Polynesian, how will that happen?" I queried.

"We'll send you to a local hair salon and get semi-permanent dye on your hair and spray it as well. You'll have to put on full body and face makeup called Texas dirt. You can shower that off every night, just don't wash your hair for the week of the show," replied one of them. HMMMMMM, okay, why not, was my answer. "Your Lieutenant Cable will be Brian Avery, who is working with you now in *My Fair Lady*."

So, I go back into rehearsal and tell the group, and they all look at me and chant "Do it, do it." I told them, "I said YES already." I'd just never seen the movie or the show live, and my castmates said, "You'll love it, you will be a beautiful Liat," and I have to admit, I was.

I will also admit that I was relieved that Carl Jablonski would no longer be the choreographer. The vibe and hostility had become so unpleasant between the female dancers and him, that we almost went to Howard and Russell, as it made us semi-miserable. It was really nobody's fault that he hadn't cast us, but he made it clear with his general attitude and lack of joy that he didn't like us too much.

So, I was happy to hear that Sheri Kirk would be our choreographer for the last three shows. She was a Sacramento native and owned a dance studio that was closed during the summer, as she wanted to perform at Music Circus.

She was skilled in all the dance forms we were doing, and simply lovely to work with. She did a wonderful job of creating my "Happy Talk" solo and mime for me, and for the rest of the show as well, and she still got to dance in the chorus. Jack Bunch did a great job directing me and Brian in our scenes together, although I was intimidated by Brian as he was twelve years older than me, and quite the Hollywood veteran, playing opposite Katharine Ross in the movie *The Graduate* and many other professional musicals.

It was a huge thrill to hear "Younger than Springtime" sung to me by him (no acting necessary), and he was more than nice to work with. I had my "hut" or the "fuck hut" as some of my castmates jokingly referred to it, up on stilts that was rushed up by the stagehands and amazingly constructed in about five minutes in the dark. There was a hanging rope ladder that I would climb up and then a few minutes later Brian would climb up, encouraged by my mother Bloody Mary, played by Evelyn Bell.

Opening night, as Brian was in the middle of singing "Younger than Springtime," Jack had directed me to run and hug Brian on the line "And when your youth and joy invade my arms." I went at him a bit too enthusiastically and almost knocked us both out of the hut, but Brian kept us from falling. The next day at preshow notes, my note from Jack was, "Linda, with your cute little apple ass, Brian would like you to not run at him so hard in the hut, or you'll both end up out of it." Brian was so professional he'd had Jack ask me!

It took me about an hour to not only warm up every night, but then to get Liat ready to make her appearance. I had what I called Liat's "Pig Pen," which was a couple of old towels Music Circus gave me for my dressing room, and they provided me with the Texas dirt, a powder make-up to apply to my body, from my feet all the way to the dance panties, then my face, neck, arms, and back, about halfway down. One of the gals would help me get it applied and then powder it down.

I had gone to a local salon and had a black semi-permanent rinse done, but it kept rubbing off on my pillowcase at night, and we had to keep spraying it nightly before each show. It really was a mess, but so worth it! I got my picture with Brian in the Sacramento Bee and a very good acting review as well, and $25 extra per performance each night!

A young couple working backstage told me I was the most beautiful woman they'd ever seen, in my sarong, a Polynesian with blue eyes. It was surprising to me since no one had ever told me I was beautiful (Al Kooper would later), and looking back it probably was the most attractive that I ever looked in a role. I was sad it only lasted one week, but the makeup and hair work were becoming a nuisance, and my hair was getting incredibly stiff from the lack of washing and all the colored spray. So, aloha nui, lovely Liat.

Musical number six was *The Student Prince.* Well, now we'll travel back in time to pre-World War I Germany. Back to the chorus go I, and become a German village girl, and a waitress in a Beer Garden.

Our stars were Linda Michelle, the amazing soprano, and John Gary as the student Prince. We did a polka in my peasant girl smock with my golden hair in two braids that reached my waist. I enjoyed the "Drinking Song," clanging metal mugs together as drunk Germans, and that was about it.

Linda Michelle was a lovely, delicate blonde that was friendly and turned me onto my vocal coach/opera coach for the next two years, Dr. Dean Verhines. He helped me achieve more vibrato and had illustrated charts of the vocal cords, and how to think of them connecting inside the throat. I was lucky to study with him.

Cast member Daniel Truhitte (he played Rolf in the movie version of *The Sound of Music*) was a Sacramento native and worked a lot for Music Circus. He was a strait-laced conservative man, and he warned us of the evils of living in Los Angles, which he'd left a few years before. "It's an evil place with everybody having sex with everybody else's wives," he cautioned, and I thought, hmmm, I will be aware of this and sort of already was, but where else would I be able to work? Not Vegas and not NYC yet.

Musical number seven was *No, No, Nanette*. This was one of the liveliest times of the summer for me. My dear grandma Frieda came down from Washington State to see me perform live for the first time in three years. We were doing a considerable amount of dancing.

Ken Berry of *Mayberry R.F.D.* and *Mama's Family* was our tap-dancing star, along with his wife Jackie Joseph, Virginia Mayo, and character actress Kathleen Freeman of numerous TV shows and Jerry Lewis movies was there for comic relief.

Best of all, my girlfriend from college, Carol "Luge" Lugenbeal, had the ingenue lead as Nanette, with her amazing soprano voice. For "Peach on the Beach," Carol, Dorothy Nichols, and I stood, center stage, on top of two-and-a-half-foot high solid beach balls, wearing ballet slippers and 20s-style bathing suits, helped up by the chorus boys, then rolling the balls with our feet in a circle and holding hands. We each got $16 a week hazard pay for that!

For this, the final show of the season, we were contracted to do two full weeks, and we actually had a day off in between. The family of our local male chorus dancer, Ron Ruge, had a party for us on our Monday night off at their lovely home in the nearby suburbs, with delicious home prepared food for the whole company. What a treat.

Towards the end of the first week, Russell and Howard asked to speak to me again. I go into their office, and they say they want a favor from me: Would I do them a favor and escort Ken Berry to the Ron Ruge party? His wife Jackie Joseph had to go back to L.A. for a work obligation on Monday, and he was without a car as he had flown to Sacramento.

"You have a Corvette, don't you?" they queried. "Yup, sure do." "So, we'll tell him you'll pick him up at 4:45. Done deal."

I had this jersey/turban outfit that I bought in Acapulco with the Bookends that was glamorous, and would get me through so many events, and this would be one of them. I was somewhat nervous about being with this big TV star, but I could do this. I picked him up at the Mansion Inn, where all of our stars stayed when doing our summer stock shows. Ken was fairly quiet but pleasant and we made some small talk driving to the suburbs. I noticed he smoked quite a bit.

We got to the party. The house was lovely, the food was GREAT, and Ken and I both mingled with different people. It was a very nice time and such a nice break, when you had to work as hard as we did, piggy backing the musicals and learning a full musical a week! Sometimes I can't believe I could do that, but it was such superb training for my TV and movie work to come.

I thanked Ron and the Ruges for the delightful party and took Ken back to the Mansion Inn. He thanked me and said, "See Ya tomorrow," for the first performance of the last week. He was an absolute gentleman, who chain smoked, at that time anyhow, and that's my Ken Berry story.

I went back to my apartment and called Al. We'd been talking two or three times a week all summer and he was finally coming up my last two days to see me. It had been about nine weeks, and I was really missing my rock star.

He meant that he hated musicals not that he hated me, but he was willing to watch me do the last one on my last day. I picked him up at the Sacramento Airport, and we immediately made love the second we got in the door. We could not get the murphy bed down fast enough. Then we went to the Mansion Inn and had a bite before the show.

As this was the closing performance, we would also be doing "Hits from the Hits" immediately after the performance. It was a bonus and an audience favorite on closing night. The producers brought back stars from the various shows over the season to perform their signature song. It lasted about a half-hour and had very little rehearsal.

Brian Avery was one of about a half dozen stars that came back for "Hits from the Hits," so I had a part with him again, despite that I was no longer his Liat. He went onstage in a blackout, and when he called to me, I ran down one of the main aisles to him. He grabbed my hand and spun me in a wide circle, and I stood and looked at him while he sang "Younger than Springtime" to me one last time. He then grabbed my hand, and we walked up an aisle together into the sunset. The aisles were always made good use of for staging, and the audience loved to be so close to us.

Al had made it thru watching *No, No, Nanette*. He chose to sit in back in the event he wanted to step out during the show. I then said my goodbyes to my castmates, many hugs and thank yous to Lewis & Young, and we went back to my murphy bed for the night.

It was great to have someone to talk to and share driving during the seven hours back to L.A. He told me that his manager, Stan Polly, had told him it was time to move out of the Blue Jay Way house, and find another rental, and time to get rid of Mickey Finn (I always felt he and the live-in maid was a bit much), so dropping both was fine by me.

So, when we got home, we'd be looking for another rental to live in. Al had a lot in storage, even furniture that he had brought from Atlanta, as the Nicky Blair house had everything, even towels and sheets.

CHAPTER FIFTEEN

THE HOUSE ON STILTS, AND MOVIES, TV, AND COMMERCIAL WORK

We found a rental within a few days after we got back about a half mile away from the Nicky Blair house, again in the hills of Hollywood. It was at the beginning of a cul de sac called Kinglet Drive. It had two floors and two bathrooms, an office/music room, spacious kitchen and living room, and it was up on stilts over a steep drop. We were assured it would make it through any severe earthquake, but I had that fear lingering in the back of my mind the entire time we lived there.

Now it was time to get a commercial agent and start auditioning for jobs in *Variety* and *The Hollywood Reporter* as that is where most musical variety jobs were cast from in the

70s. You didn't need an agent yet, but you had to be wary of most acting jobs in those papers, as many were bogus.

I auditioned for a great commercial agency and got accepted to Sonja Warren Brandon's Commercials Unlimited, run and owned by the gorgeous Sonja. However, I had to take a commercial acting class, as auditioning for and filming commercials were very different than other forms of film work.

So, I took a six-week course from an older casting director, Maxine Anderson's Commercial Way class, and I really needed it. A heads up for ANY actor looking to book commercials: You must know how to slate, look at and talk directly to the camera for spokesperson style commercials, and when not to look at camera for multi-person commercials, staying on the mark, and how to "button" or "tag" the endings.

I auditioned for some mostly dancing or singing jobs in films or TV shows. I did not want to work as a Bookend again for a while, if ever. I went to an audition for a movie looking for singers, dancers, and variety talent in their 20s, and I believe the ad said, "There may be nudity required for some parts, but not all." It was at the Masonic Temple on Hollywood Blvd. It had several large studios with sprung wood floors, which I'd been to many times, and all of the auditions there were legit.

I walked into the large audition room with my now "real" headshot, resumé, sheet music, and always my dance bag, full of dance shoes, mostly Capezio heels and heeled tap shoes, ballet shoes, etc.

Up front was a table with four men: Bruce Kimmel, star, writer, and co-director, Lloyd Gordon, choreographer, Mark Haggard, co-director, and Jack Reeves, producer. So, I'm auditioning for Bruce's film *The First Nudie Musical.* I also recognized a newly made friend who I'd done a commercial audition with playing sisters, Susan Buckner, who would become my lifelong friend until she passed away in 2023.

She was from Burien, and I was from Bremerton, a ferry boat ride away! She was very beautiful with the best legs I'd ever seen. We got our street clothes off, a pair of jeans, over leotards and tights, and put our jazz shoes on. Lloyd Gordon gave us a jazz combination first and then for those of us who could tap a relatively simple tap combination. Susan and I made the cut for both and were offered a job on the spot.

The first was supporting dancer/actors as sex workers at "Wanda's Brothel," fully clothed. Also, the finale tap dance number, that would be in top hat, tails, bow tie, and tap shoes, the rest of the female form visible and quite nude. Susan said yes to the hooker part, but no to the nude tap dance.

I said yes to the hooker part and then asked questions about the tap dance: Could I wear a wig to rehearsals and for the shoot? Could I change my name on the credits to something other than my real and union name and the answer to both was YES!!! So, okay, I'll accept the role as one of the tap dancing "vaginas." I was a natural born rebel who enjoyed challenges, but back then nudity could be a negative for an entertainer's career, unlike even twenty years later. Then, in the 2000s, it was pretty much no big deal, as long as it wasn't hardcore porn. So, I had two parts I booked.

I rushed home to the stilts house to tell Al about my new job that would start in about a week. It was my first movie and my first spoken screen line as well. Then I told him about the tap dance, and he thought that it was so cool and so brave of me to do. I was going to wear a shitty, cheap wig for the entire tap experience and we needed to come up with a name for me, so we came up with "Kathy Wiglett". It was my sister's first name, and of course, referenced the wig disguise.

We rehearsed and filmed the sex worker number first. Our costumes were outrageous for "Honey Wat'cha Doin' Tonight." I was in a gray afro with hot pants and long eyelashes with glitter. I LOVED this song and Bruce Kimmel was the only male and star of the number, as he was our reluctant virgin "John." It also featured Susan Buckner and Cindy Ashley who I had danced with several times in my career.

Then a couple of weeks went by, and we shot the finale with the nude tap dance. I did wear my wig and had people call me "Kathy." There were male tappers in this routine as well and none of the females were in the previous number with me, so it worked out fine.

We rehearsed with clothes on, of course, until shoot day. We "tapping vaginas" were only concerned about one thing: What to do with the tampon string if we were on our periods? We figured out quickly we'd just have to push it up as far as we could and hope for the best. Fortunately, when the shoot day arrived, none of us were on our periods, yay!

It was awesome having Cindy Williams as our female star, surreal actually, as she was a huge TV star on *Laverne and Shirley*. She played the producer's secretary, and there was no nudity involved at all for her. She was also extraordinarily down to earth as a star.

One day after lunch we were in the ladies' room together, and she was brushing her teeth at one of the sinks. When I came out of the stall, I said, "How smart of you to bring a toothbrush, I'll have to start doing that," and she replied, "Would you like to borrow it?" (The toothbrush.) WOW! I politely said something like "Oh no, that's so nice of you, but I'll bring my own, tomorrow," and was impressed by her and will never forget her kindness.

We shot the finale successfully although when I finally saw the end product, I looked sort of nervous facially, but my dancing was fine. And really, all you could see was our pubic hair patch, our "bush" as we referred to it back then, not even our boobs or our butts. I was also asked to record the tap sounds with choreographer Lloyd Gordon, as I had the strongest tap skills. We stood on a large, hollow wooden box with a microphone underneath it, and headphones on. This is the way it was done for many movies and TV shows back then. It was an honor to do it.

The movie came out and it was a pretty big success, even making it into the top grossing films of 1977 in *Variety*. This year, 2025, we celebrate the 50th anniversary of the actual shooting in 1975. It came out on Blu-ray in 2015, and I went to a screening and Q&A for that event. 50 years later, it's still a cult classic. Bruce Kimmel is still my buddy and I'm always so happy for his success. He still calls me "Wiglett," which cracks me up.

Life was zooming along, and I booked my first commercial during this time period as well. It was a national for McDonalds as a counter girl called, "The French Fry Kid." Unfortunately, it did not run. They have to run to make the residuals, and sometimes they don't. I found out later through my agents that they got a master shot with another business in it and had to scrap the ad. I made "day rate", which was $1,200, and still the best money an actor can make (per second) and why you do commercials.

Ray Anthony called me in the middle of November and asked if I could help him out and work three weeks, from early December to right after New Years, as one of the other gals had to spend the holidays with her mother who was very ill. Al had to go back East for the same three weeks to produce Lynyrd Skynyrd's third album, *Nuthin' Fancy*, so he'd be gone, too, at that time. I thought why not, we had no pets, and didn't worry about getting robbed—about the only thing they could get was records and guitars.

The booking was at the Golden Nugget in Reno, and I had never been there. I thought I could handle the holidays on the road, which I had never done yet, but at least it was with my Bookend girlfriends. Reno was sort of gross back then, with not a lot to do, but it had some snow. We went to see the movie, *Earthquake*, which was the only movie playing in town. The movie had a man standing on the balcony of a house on stilts, eating a piece of fried chicken, as it collapses. Great huh? Well, lesson learned, there's no place like home for the holidays.

CHAPTER SIXTEEN

WORKING ON THE SMOTHERS BROTHERS AND "OTHERS"

I booked a commercial for Japan at the end of January. When you did commercials for foreign countries, they were referred to as "buyouts" because it was too difficult for the country to monitor the commercial for residuals, and it was allowed by SAG and AFTRA, which I had joined in 1974. Since I was already a member of AEA, the union for Actors and Stage Managers, it only cost me $150 to join SAG, and another $75 to join AFTRA. That's so crazy in today's world —SAG/AFTRA is $3000, and you do not get a break if you're AEA, which I think is totally unfair considering they are sister entertainment unions, but not my call.

Anyway, the commercial was for Nikki Whiskey, called "Have a Nikki Night," and it was shot in a silent movie style in black and white. It had Keystone Kops coming out of a manhole, with others following the cops out.

My character was a white swan ballerina who came out of the manhole and pas de bourréed away with white swan arms, sur la point, as I still took ballet classes from time-to-time en pointe. It was fun and only took a day to shoot for $500 flat.

I finally got a call from Walter Painter to come to an audition for the 1975 edition of *The Smothers Brothers Show*, the naughty, liberal boys of TV comedy who most of us just fucking LOVED. It was at NBC in Burbank. Oh boy! My main goal of my career was to dance with the stars that I grew up watching on TV. I was bound and determined to get this, and I nailed the audition, not that I needed to, as Walter was in my corner.

It was the end of January 1975, and I did my first TV show dancing to "Mr. Bojangles," while the Smothers Brothers sang, and the eight of us dancers did a stylized dance during the instrumental section. I was nervous as hell as we had a live audience and were on national TV in front of millions of people. Some of my senior dancers were there with me, including Karen Lauren, Lorraine Fields, Rava Daly, and assistant choreographer, Sandy Roveta. They were so supportive that I would be eternally grateful to them.

The guest star that week was Mason Williams, playing his hit song "Classical Gas." He played it on a see-through, clear plastic guitar, filled with water and two goldfish inside. It kept leaking, but they finally got a take.

Two weeks later, we did a crazy square dance production number that was such a blast that it wasn't like working at all. You can still see it on YouTube. It featured the entire cast of *The Smothers Brothers Show*, including Pat Paulson, Jennifer Warne and all the dancers.

Before we started taping that production number, Tommy Smothers came up to me, grabbed my face in both hands, gave me a huge toilet plunger kiss on the lips and ran away. I was speechless and thrilled for him to do so, and I guess he liked me?

We went and grabbed people from the audience towards the end of the song and danced with them on the soundstage. My chosen partner was a long-haired guy who may have been drunk or stoned, but he was sort of out of my control, and I laughed my ass off knowing this would be on national TV.

The final episode I did for the Smothers Brothers was with Ray Charles guest starring, and there were only four dancers hired for this one, at least that I can recall. When I walked into our rehearsal hall at NBC, Ray Charles was sitting just to the right of the door. I was honestly starstruck for the first time in my life. I could not stop staring and good thing he was blind, as it might've been rude if he could see me. Walter choreographed a sexy dance for us, and then it cut to the four girl dancers on our stomachs, doing knee bends on his baby grand piano.

We had very cute costumes with a low back and poofy round feathers covering our cute little butts. It was also my first experience with a body makeup lady. What a pleasant experience that was! She put make up on our backs, arms, and necks with a warm sponge, and it was so soothing. This lady said to me, "You know who you look like, don't You?"

My reply was, "No not really." She said, "Ann-Margret." That really made my day, my week, my YEAR! Ann-Margret was the inspirational person in my life that unknowingly mentored me. We were both Scandinavian, she more than me, and Svenska, as I was one-third Norsky, so perhaps that explained it?

Apparently, the director had a drinking problem and instead of shooting over our poofy feather butts to a direct shot of Ray's face, he shot our feather butts, missing Ray's face entirely! Disappointingly, the entire production number was cut from the episode, and that was the last one I did with the Smothers Brothers. But what a wonderful first TV series job. I will always love that, and my Brothers Smothers.

One afternoon at the end of January, Al comes home with a 3/4" videotape and says, "Come upstairs and watch this band with me. A&M Records wants to record and handle them, but nobody will produce them. They are a performance art rock band called The Tubes, and they are supposed to have quite the show." Our video tape player was in our bedroom sitting on top of a chest of drawers so we could rent videos and watch TV in bed.

I can't remember what song The Tubes opened their show with, but the lead singer was very animated. They also had a male dancer, Kenny Ortega, and a female dancer and sometimes singer, Re Styles, two guitar players, a bass guitar player, an organ player and a drummer, Prairie Prince. Their songs were catchy and on the humorous side, with props and costume changes by the lead singer, Fe Waybill. Two of their outstanding songs were "Don't Touch Me There," with Fe and Re on a real motorcycle, and "Mondo Bondage," with Fe in bondage gear, wearing a leather mask, and leather chap type pants, with his bare butt crack showing in back and a black whip that he dragged around and cracked.

Everyone's favorite was Fe, as a Rod Stewart lookalike named Quay Lude, with his white pineapple hairdo, white skintight Lycra unitard, and 12-inch platform boots that he could barely walk in, singing "White Punks on Dope." It was a song about rich Hollywood youth spending their movie star parents' money, and teenage drug addiction. At the end, he falls off his platforms and angels sing and help him to heaven in a big instrumental finale. FAB-U-LOUS!

I looked at Al and said, "YOU WILL PRODUCE THEM! YOU'LL PRODUCE THEM FOR ME!!!" "Okay, okay," was Al's reply, and he did.

He worked very hard on the enhanced recorded versions of The Tubes first album, with lots of added arrangements and sound effects. It was released in March of 1975, fifty years ago this year.

The Tubes started touring and it was sooo fun to see them in person, and when they came to L.A., we saw them several times. Of course, I was their biggest fan. They came up to the house on stilts to hang out once, and my sister was visiting from San Diego. It was cute to see Fe flirting with Kathy, but that was about as far as it went. They would've made a cute couple.

The Tubes went on a BIG tour, and it helped with album sales, but it never got very high on the charts as they toured the world, mostly Europe. Their stage act of course was a huge, huge hit, as it should be, and they will always be one of my favorite live bands. As I write this in 2025, they are still touring sporadically.

Al had come back from making Lynyrd Skynyrd's third album *Nuthin' Fancy* totally burned out. The band had really made it now, and they also had become out of control party boys. They had been touring constantly and had done very little song writing, and it was tremendously hard to get enough songs recorded and pulled together in the two weeks they had booked at WEB1V studios in Atlanta. The "Swamp Boys" as I referred to them, also had an entourage of friends and groupies with them which was constantly disruptive, as well as the whiskey and weed and who knows what else.

The only song from that album that I liked was "Whiskey Rock-a-Roller" that was a shuffle and very representative of them. Things got so bad, particularly with Ronnie's drinking and temper, that after Ronnie beat him up, guitarist Ed King just snuck away to the airport and ran away from the tour they had just started after the album's conclusion.

They had developed a bad reputation as a violent, hard drinking band. Al told them that he was glad to have worked with them. They made a lot of money and achieved fame, but he was done as their producer. They came into town in April of '75. They were touring and promoting their latest and third album for MCA. We weren't going to go and see them, which I found sad, but I don't think Al felt entirely safe around them at that point in time.

A pretty, bodacious girlfriend of mine, Coleen Hinton, had asked me if she could meet them. She was single and liked rockers, although she was not a groupie. I had already made friends with Gary Rossington when we hung out with them. He was only a year older than me and somewhat shy and sweet. So, I invited them over to hang the afternoon of the first show and see if there was any chemistry there, and ... there was.

Gary invited her to the show that night and they hit it off. I had to admit that I missed seeing Skynyrd live, and I never did again as fate would have it, but Coleen and Gary saw each other a few times when Gary and the band came to town.

After the release of The Tubes album titled *The Tubes*, A&M records was pleased with what Al did and asked if he would produce a solo album for guitarist, Nils Lofgren, who had also been a member of Neil Young's band Crazy Horse for a while.

Nils was this cute young man who was a genius at playing lead guitar, who could also sing. He didn't have a great voice, but pleasant for rock music. There was no time to record in the ever-popular Record Plant, but there was Record Plant North up in Sausalito. Sly Stone had a customized recording studio there that he rented out and it was available. The Record Plant also included a house with several bedrooms, bathrooms, and a creepy looking hot tub that looked like there had been many bodies in it engaging in various sexual activities that came as part of the "package" for bands, artists, their significant others, while recording in Sausalito.

It was decided that that was what they would do for about two weeks, maybe three. Nice for them! I'd just stay in L.A., take various classes which I continued to do throughout my career, and hold down the fort. We were trying to have one or the other of us not go on the road at the same time anymore, and I was attempting to work in town more anyway.

The plan was, towards the end of the recording of the album, I'd fly up and spend the weekend with my boyfriend. Al and I had been talking on the phone during the session in Sausalito. He had a severe problem with his recording engineer, who was coked up all the time and he had to replace him with another engineer from L.A. Other than that, the recording of *Cry Tough* was going smoothly, and Nils was easy to get along with.

I fly up to Sausalito, and somebody from the studio and the Record Plant house picks me up and brings me to the recording studio. I walk in the door to Sly Stone's studio and yowza, wowza!! It is covered from floor to ceiling with red shag carpeting, except for the sound board in the middle of the room, and the chairs.

There is a big tank of nitrous oxide on the floor in front of the sound board, and Al motions for me to come and lay down with him. So, I do, and we both share hits from it together and look into each other's eyes. The nitrous has an orgasmic quality for me, it felt very sexual, and was like breathing in sex.

Next, Nils comes in, as he'd been outside in the parking lot shooting hoops with Bob Edwards, the new engineer.

They had to put some finishing touches on a track before workday's end. Nils and Bob are both very congenial and the four of us went to dinner before going back to the Record Plant house. I really liked the place with all the knotty pine on the inside that had a great pine scent to it.

The next day was to be the last day working on the album, putting finishing touches on certain tracks, and the last day of nitrous, damn it! But it was a strong gas and could be dangerous, and Al could feel it affecting his ulcers.

About halfway through the day, Sly came through the hallway and into his studio with what looked like a bodyguard, or at least a big burley friend. He was kind of stumbling and had a shit eatin' grin on his face, wearing a fur coat with a lot of gold bling, and a huge 'fro.

He stayed for just a few minutes, seemingly stoned on something, as he didn't seem to be able to say much and then just split, stumbling out. It was just classic Sly. He had a hard time making it to his own concerts because of various drug issues. What a waste of talent, as his music was so danceable.

The final day we said our goodbyes and flew back to L.A. Al had produced five tracks on the album, and Nils was to add another five from a previous recording session, and that would become *Cry Tough*. It was not a big hit in the U.S., but it won the Silver Award in Great Britain, as it was more popular there. I still like the album and it reminds me of getting high on nitrous!

It is May now, and I haven't booked much since *The Smothers Brothers Show*. I was collecting unemployment, which was a way of life in the entertainment industry, a safety net if you will, when not working, as we were basically all gig workers. You still had to physically go to the unemployment office down in the dregs of Hollywood and show up in person. There were no dog poop laws yet, and people in that general area just let their dogs shit all over the pavement and not pick it up! It was filthy and disgusting and I literally jete'd over the piles of poop that were all over the sidewalks, to stay in shape.

It was amusing to be in the Hollywood office, as many a famous actor would be in and collecting what they did pay into. Dustin Hoffman was one that stands out in my mind, but there were so many TV actors I cannot even recall everyone. Of course, I'd run into some of my fellow cast members, as well. And then there's that famous story about Ann Miller, the tap dancer/actress in many a movie musical, that filled out her occupation on her UE form as STAR, not actress, dancer or singer, just STAR.

Stan Polly and I had a talk and we both agreed that it was time for Al to buy a house and not rent. He was just throwing money away and had no real property to show for it. Our next project was house hunting. We started looking in the Hollywood Hills area, as Beverly Hills was a bit out of our price range.

After looking at about ten homes in a little over a week, we came upon one that was just "us"! It was on Dalegrove Drive, just off Coldwater Canyon, on a side street cul de sac, going up into the hills. It was owned by a man living with his teenage son (he was divorced). He had a fun personality and owned a DeLorean! We learned he was a writer for the TV series *Happy Days* and was very nice to deal with.

The house was so pleasing from outside. It was a ranch-style house with a rectangle swimming pool beside it. The exterior of the house was all wood with an unfinished-looking orange-brown color, with red brick columns holding up the covered walkway to a rec room with a sliding glass door, with the main front entry farther down.

About halfway down the length of the building was a second floor held up by another set of brick columns. We had never seen anything quite like it. It had an attached double garage, but also room in front of the house and driveway, with parking for three more cars. It had a long rec room downstairs at the entrance, a long kitchen, a half-bath downstairs, a living room/dining room, and an alcove off the dining room.

Upstairs was one bedroom with a fucking fabulous view of Coldwater Canyon out a huge window, a large bathroom with a jacuzzi tub, a shower stall, and his and hers sinks. Asking price in 1976: $135,000. Al offered the seller $140,000 on the spot, to take it off the market! It will be named "Freebird Mansion" after the obvious, and we were thrilled.

We, however, were not going to be able to move in for a while, as there was escrow to go through, and Al had big plans for the interior that needed more style and drama. My man had a vision, and it turned out spectacularly.

He hired some wood workers from Australia who customized the upstairs bedroom, built a long bunkbed in the rec room that would serve as our guest bed that Al named the "balling ally". Should I have been suspicious? He also rebuilt the spiral staircase that went up to our wooden king-sized bed, that I can't begin to describe. He had a rotating "dry cleaning" closet put in the bedroom for his exotic clothes, while mine got squished into a small closet off the master bath upstairs. Well ... he was the "Rock Star," wasn't he?

Now I hadn't worked much at all since the *Smothers* show, and I was sort of running out of unemployment. I know I was with a millionaire, but even so, I prided myself on some financial independence and still do to this day.

My husbands or boyfriends have never given me a credit card to just go for it with clothes, jewelry, etc. I had been spending quality time with my man and enjoying it, but it was time to go back to work. So, Ray Anthony called and asked if I would do two months in Honolulu, headlining the showroom at the glamorous and very pink Royal Hawaiian Hotel on Kalākaua Avenue on the Waikiki strip.

I ran it by Al, and he said it was logical, and we would probably move soon after I returned. More perfect moving karma!

Off to Hawaii I go with my Bookend girlfriends. I shared an apartment off the Alamu Canal with three other cast members in a rather cramped apartment, but we could use all the facilities at the Royal Hawaiian, including the pool, beachfront, and even the showers.

We performed a show a night for six nights with one day off. I still loved Hawaii, but as time went on, I developed what they called "Island Fever" toward the end of the two months. Besides, I missed Al.

I behaved like a local, riding public transit, picking mangos up off the ground and taking them home to eat, going to the swap meet inside Diamond Head crater, and buying bags of Macadamia nuts. But perhaps the most bizarre thing that happened when I was there was running into my high school sociology teacher, Mr. Gary Anderson, on a remote jungle road by a friend's house on the North Shore!

I had befriended a local jeweler, Paul Cross, and his girlfriend, who had invited me to their house on a day off. I went for a change of pace. We went out on some surfboards to just play around until Paul informed us that he'd heard there were hammerhead sharks seen in the area. We paddled the surfboards quickly back to shore!

We started to get hungry, and Paul told us he'd treat us to Shabu Shabu back in Honolulu, so we got dressed, but Paul's beater little Datsun had starter issues, so the three of us pushed it up the sloped driveway so he could run it downhill to start it. We neared the top of the driveway and ... there was my social studies teacher, GARY ANDERSON, just standing there. It was surreal, and we both looked like we'd seen a ghost!

"Mr. Anderson, what are you doing here?!" I yelled.

"What are YOU doing here Linda?" he yelled back, and we both were laughing hard by now. Our reply to each other was "Visiting friends!"

I invited him to see my show at the Royal Hawaiian, but I don't think he ever came. I did tell him he was one of my favorite teachers in high school and thanked him for making us read *The American Way of Death*, a book about consumer trickery that served me my entire life. We had to get going, and I never saw him again, but what a weird coincidence!

At the end of the two months, I couldn't wait to get back to the homeland for so many reasons, and the gig went off without any hassle from Ray, as he'd given up on me by now. Al picks me up at LAX in one of his newer cars, a Cadillac compact four-door, turquoise and white. It was cute, but it sort of reminded me of a pimp car.

He had gotten rid of the Silver Cloud Rolls and the Citroen Maserati. He'd also bought a moss-green Mercedes, and I still had the Corvette. We went back to the house on stilts but did not make love. Al had come down with a case of his chronic herpes simplex which he'd had for years and was good enough to not want to pass it onto me. So, we had some of Al's chicken soup and then headed over to our home-to-be, which was still a work in progress, as it was about a week to ten days out.

There, we meet the two Australian carpenters and also Lenny Bruce's widow, the former stripper Honey Bruce, who was about 50 years old, and her daughter Kitty who were friends of the carpenters. It turns out Al is infatuated with Honey. When Al was 16 years old, he snuck into see Lenny Bruce at Carnegie Hall. Al didn't shy away from sexual humor, he loved it, the saltier the better. It was such an oddity that the carpenters were friends with the Bruce women.

I was starstruck with Honey as well, Hot Honey Harlowe, who was portrayed in the movie *Lenny* directed by Bob Fosse. Young Kitty, approximately 18, kept doing Fosse hands and the walk and talking about Bob, but she was not a dancer. Honey was still attractive with red hair, but time and drugs had left their mark on her skin, and she did look her age. Her figure was still pretty good, and she was romantically involved with one of the carpenters. They were all staying in the house in sleeping bags and air mattresses as there was no furniture in there yet except the bed, and "Balling Ally" with a mattress so they also slept there.

We went home and I unpacked, did laundry etc., and the next day I jumped piles of dog poop to file for unemployment.

Al and I also went carpet and furniture shopping for Freebird Mansion, and the next week was spent packing our clothes, household goods, etc., and taking some to the house. I loved hanging out with Honey, especially, and I hated seeing her go. She made me my first pair of feather earrings, which was a hobby for her, and she and Kitty were also painting the kitchen and small bathroom for Al. Honey was always so incredibly good-natured, so happy.

We also had a week in between moving into Freebird Mansion and the end of our house on stilts lease, so we rented a bungalow at the Beverly Hills Hotel, which was just beautiful. We ate at the Polo Lounge twice a day. If you've never been in the Polo Lounge, do go sometime—if the walls could talk! It was always, at least at that time, chock full of stars and their agents or managers dining, drinking, and making lots of deals. It was classic Beverly Hills, the epitome of "A list" Hollywood. Before we stayed in the bungalow, we would frequently meet Al's manager Stan Polly there for a breakfast of lox and bagels and for coffee talk. I just loved that!

We moved in and it took us a couple of weeks to pull the place together. Al chose the furniture and white shag carpet under the white baby grand in the alcove, and all his records went on shelves around that. The living room also had an area white shag carpet, with a white conversation L-shaped couch. The house had very lovely hardwood floors and we wanted to show them off. The living room had one of the first large screen TVs and state-of-the-art stereo equipment.

Al bought a pool table and a pinball machine for the game room and lined the walls of the game room with his guitars, including the Fender Strat that Jimi Hendrix gave him at the Monterey Pop Festival that he stage managed in '67. There was also a Hammond organ in front of the wall. We had very little artwork on the walls or family pictures; it just didn't need it. The entire house was just a showstopper for the many celebs that would eventually visit, and our friends and family as well.

Time to start working again, but I was not going to audition for road shows, as I wanted to enjoy my new digs. And it was time for pets!! I was given a puppy at a commercial audition, a little black mix that another actress begged me to take, but I'd never had a puppy before, so I didn't know what I was doing. Al named it Bozo as it was a clumsy little boy. I took it to get shots and fixed and fed it twice a day and tried to do the best I could, but Al wanted him to stay outside, so we got it a doghouse for the big backyard.

The backyard was a large spare lot with dirt, and dead grass and weeds but fenced in. It had a lemon tree and kumquat tree to one side, but other than that, no flowers, no care and a waste except for the pets.

The owner and his son also left me their white cat, a full-grown fellow named Drooling John as he drooled when you petted him. He was, unfortunately, an indoor/

outdoor cat who liked to bring us presents like lizards and mice. We had him for a couple of months and then poof, he just disappeared. It was thought that the coyotes were his untimely end. Although we'd never actually seen any, they were there.

I auditioned for Walter, who was doing *The Tony Orlando and Dawn Show*, and the one episode I did was guest-starring Freddie Prinze. We were a production number where the girl dancers were street hookers and Freddie was our pimp, and I believe Freddie sang as we all danced around him, trying to look our sexy hooker best for him.

When we were on a break one day, I passed Freddie on the payphone in the hall of NBC and overheard him talking to his therapist. I lingered just a bit, but he sounded so depressed. Hmmm. It made me concerned, but I didn't know him, so I stayed out of it. The episode aired a week later and our production number with Freddie was completely cut! I was so disappointed because it was only my second TV series, and of course, it was working with Freddie.

I phoned Walter up the next day, and he said that the director was the same alcoholic that was used on *The Smothers Brothers Show* who'd shot the feathers on our butts and not Ray Charles. Walter said that the director shot Freddie under the street light that was part of our pimp/hooker set, but instead of shooting Freddie, he just shot Freddie's hands adjusting his cufflinks, which was a bit Freddie was given, but not Freddie, so we come dancing out to nobody with our feather boas and miniskirts on, and it was just not salvageable. One had to wonder why this director was getting hired at all for network TV shows, but apparently, he was not hired again after that one.

About three weeks later, the news came on and reported that Freddie had taken his own life. The show biz community, me included, was devasted hearing this.

That episode of *Tony Orlando and Dawn* was his final work before he died.

Next, I auditioned for Jaime Rodgers for *The Sonny and Cher Show.* Jaime was this stocky little Puerto Rican dancer/choreographer, who was one of the two choreographers who were known as sexual harassers of female dancers in Hollywood in the 70s. He was well known for his work as one of the Sharks in the movie *West Side Story,* and for co-choreographer of the famous '68 comeback special for Elvis Presly where he and Claude Thompson created the most athletic dance work on TV of that era.

He was hired a lot and worked a lot despite the the knowledge that he was a well-known stalker of pretty female dancers. It's odd, too, that he and the other male chorographer/harasser were both married, and both to other female dancers who assisted choreographers or still danced themselves. The wives must've turned a blind eye to the situation.

For this episode, Jaime hired all blonde female dancers, that included a couple of girlfriends of mine, including Susan Buckner, who was my good buddy. It was discussed by us, away from Jaime, that we should be aware that he may try to get us up to his "office" to discuss our careers, his apparent method of choice to be alone with a naïve young dancer.

Our episode was with the guest star Raymond Burr of *Perry Mason* fame. I thought it was sort of an odd choice, but it worked out well. As I walked into the rehearsal hall that morning to begin, I heard a voice that sounded like Raymond Burr to the right of me as I went through the door, but it had an added lateral lisp or as some called it "S's for days."

There to my right sat Raymond conversing with the director about his role on the episode. WOW, what a shockaroonie to hear this masculine man with this gay lisp, but I found out soon from others on the set that sure 'nuff, he preferred men and had a male partner. I was amazed how he could control his voice when acting and completely rid himself of that speech impediment.

I also learned that Sonny and Cher were separated, and Cher was expecting Greg Allman's baby. He was the new man in her life, although I don't think they were married yet. Despite this situation, it was not a tense set. Cher had a female assistant who looked like her, and who was always by her side.

Cher never made eye contact with any of us or as much as looked our way, she kept her distance at a table away from the supporting cast and did not want any sort of conversation from us. I would have loved to have told her how much I admired her, but no way. People always ask me about her and working with her and I have next to nothing to say about her.

The female dancers had two different parts in this episode, as sketch actresses and in the musical production number. We did a sketch starring Sonny as Sam Spade, a detective along the lines of Inspector Clouseau, who is a bumbling idiot but solves cases. Cher was the other female lead, but her part was brief.

I had the best non-speaking role of the four or five blondes, a nice spot with Sonny. He would come over to the bar in the Casbah Club and I was sitting on a stool by myself, looking really sexy in my up do and 40s outfit as it was set in the 40s, a la *Casablanca.* He ordered his usual drink as I looked at him longingly and tried to get his attention by running my hands on his shoulders, but he shot his drink, ignored me, and walked away.

We were rehearsing this for a couple of days, and he says to me, "Hey, you're pretty cute, how'd you like to come to dinner with me?" and he was serious. Now, I wasn't much attracted to Sonny, and I knew the situation with

Cher, but hell ... he was the star of the show so kid gloves, kid gloves.

I said, "Oh, that's so nice of you to ask, I'm so flattered, but I have a boyfriend, in fact like you, he's a songwriter and singer. His name is Al Kooper, and I live with him. Do you know who he is?" "No," was his reply. "So, I can't, but thanks so much!" was my reply, and he seemed fine with that, and we did a good scene with no negative vibes.

Our production number was called "The Monstrel Minstrel Show" and it should've been the Halloween show, but it wasn't. It starred Sonny, Cher, and Raymond Burr as three creepy vampires, and the rest of us on benches below them, dressed as all the other scary creatures, mainly walking around, changing places on the benches, as the three of them made a series of ghoulish jokes.

I was a skeleton, Susan Buckner was a witch, one was a werewolf (we did have a few males in the chorus that week), one was Frankenstein, Frankenstein's bride, a ghost, the mummy, etc. Our makeup took many makeup artists two hours to get all of us done.

As we walked around, we mostly did posture and arm movements that suited our characters, and then we all sat down to sing our minstrel song. We had been sent home to memorize it, although it was done to a recorded track with lip-syncing. "The sun goes down, the moon comes up, dagger in the back and poison in the cup. Uh huh, Dracula, it's so neat to beat your feet in the Mississippi mud," and so on, and a few more silly lines. It was a blast, and very easy!

I was headed out the door after taping day, and Jaime is behind me, and he says, "Hey Linda, can you come up to my office, I'd like to discuss your career?!" To be forewarned is to be forearmed and I said, "Oh Jaime, how nice of you but I have a planning dinner tonight with my fiancé about our wedding."

Jaime mumbled something under his breath (he was a well-known mumbler, as well as a sexual stalker) but he just said "Okay, bye." Now the wedding thing wasn't entirely false, as Al had offered to marry me about two weeks after we began living together. He simply said, "I'll marry you if you want me to," but I gently said, "I'm too young for that at twenty-one, maybe later when I'm older, my love." And of course, there was the philandering issue, which I truly tried not to think about too much, but it was there.

Next, I auditioned for a rare job as a female replacement dancer for *The Carol Burnett Show*. Carol Burnett had a wildly popular weekly variety show that had a group of a dozen contracted male and female dancers—six men and six women. They were all good dancers, sketch actors, and some gymnasts, and all tap dancers as well.

One of the female dancers had come down with a serious illness and had to retire from dancing altogether, so Ernie Flatt was looking for one female dancer to replace her. It was a "cattle call" audition at CBS studios with about 300 female dancers answering the call from the ad in *Variety*.

Ernie had his assistant George give us a fast-footed combination, a la "Ernie style" that we all learned together, then he separated us into groups of eight, did it twice with the row switch, followed by thank yous to many groups of us. Only about twenty-five of us were kept, and yes, I was one! We were told that no one would be chosen that day, but if you were selected, you'd receive a phone call from George.

A few days later, I was at CBS auditioning for another show, but a much smaller audition. We were across the hall from Carol's studio, dancing hard when two of the Burnett dancers, Stan Mazin and Bobbie Bates, and George appeared in our open doorway watching us. When we had a short break, they motioned to me to come over to the door.

"Are you working next week?" George asked.

"No, I am not" I replied.

"Do we have your phone number? I'll give you a call tonight with your schedule," he said, and then they went back to their rehearsal.

Was I over the moon or what? My goodness God Almighty, the BURNETT SHOW!!! I also booked the TV show I was auditioning for, *The Brady Bunch Variety Hour* but that would not start for about three weeks. I rushed home and told Al, and I was so HAPPY.

George called me and told me my call time, a five-day typical schedule for a variety TV show, with a fitting with costumer Bob Mackie at the end of the week. Bob Mackie, too, was incredible and such a nice man, and my costume was going to be gorgeous—a hot pink satin skirt and crop top.

Day One of rehearsal, I walked into the rehearsal studio, and to the right of me standing and speaking to the director was Mr. Cool himself, Sammy Davis Jr.! We would be dancing behind him as he sang a mashup of the Doobie Brothers' "Taking it to the Streets" into "What Kind of Fool Am I?"

Sammy had a large head and a skinny body and was only about 5'5". He was smoking one of his many cigarettes that day, but it was his left hand that caught my interest. His baby fingernail was about an inch long and painted red. It was his "coke" finger, so he would not need a spoon. I'd only heard of that but never seen one.

We were assigned partners by Ernie and placed with the five other couples. My partner was Stan Mazin, a long time Burnett dancer and a handsome man, about 5'10". He was a great dancer and a caring and wonderful human being who had helped me get this job, along with female Burnett dancer, Bobbie Bates. What an honor from both. It was a partner dance with the woman's arm on the man's shoulder, with the man facing backwards and the female forward, and then we would switch, the man would face front, but the woman would just switch her arm to the other shoulder. Sounds strange, but it had a kind of a Latin look to it, along with Ernie's signature fast footwork.

I was treated very nicely by the Burnett dancers, especially Stan, Bobbie, and Sandy Johnson. On the second day of rehearsal, we got a real treat. Harvey Korman and Tim Conway came in and performed their sketch for the week in front of us, and Tim, of course, cracked Harvey up. On the third day, we pretty much had our dance behind Sammy down pat, and I started feeling a bit off. I felt like my dance pick up (how fast you catch on and remember the chorography) had been on the slow side all week, although Ernie's fast style was new to me, and quite unique. When I went home, I started to feel even worse. I had some of Al's chicken soup, but I felt like shit, and took a quickie shower, and went and laid down. But that didn't help for long, I was up and barfing my guts out. And this continued through the night with intermittent naps.

Fortunately for me, Ernie gave us the next day off, as we had the dance down and had no sketch work that week. I was still so weak and sick. It was a neuro virus or as some refer to it, stomach flu. Al called Ernie Flatt, told him who he was and said, "Linda can't come in tomorrow, she's very sick and weak, throwing up all night long!" And Ernie said, "She has to come in, I have nobody to replace her, and it's taping day. Get her to a doctor and tell them the true situation, they can help."

Luckily our doctors were "Dr. Feelgoods", and they had Linda Ronstadt, Rod Stewart and us as patients. The show must go on, so Dr. Cantor gave me a shot of speed and a prescription for Ritalin for the morning. I actually went to sleep later that night even with the shot. I got up early, had my Ritalin dose, and drove myself to CBS.

I was still sort of weak and green as I got into hair and makeup, and then Bob Mackie poured me into my stunning Bob Mackie gown. We went to our little elevated stage on the soundstage about a foot off the ground. We marked the dance once with Sammy and his red fingernail (thank God he wasn't smoking), then playback began, and we did the dance musical number behind Mr. Entertainment IN ONE TAKE! I had made a small booboo turn, but Stan knew I was slightly out of it and whipped me around real fast, so it wasn't noticeable.

I sat on the side of our platform stage as playback was checked by Ernie and our director, who announced, "That's a wrap," which had never happened to me so far with a taped production number. The Burnett show had it down to a science! We were all going towards the dressing rooms, yay, and Carol Burnett came in from another studio and said, "Not so fast everybody, Sammy is going to do a show for us across the hall in Studio 29, so as soon as you get out of costume, come over and have a seat, you don't want to miss this." As sick as I still felt, oh no I didn't.

We all truck on over to Studio 29 across the hall, take our seats and Sammy and a piano player do a fantastic one-man show for about forty-five minutes for the cast and crew. It was unforgettable, including a lot of his hits, and a little bit of tap as well. It was such a nice way to end a challenging forty-eight hours for me.

I never got asked back to do another show, as I didn't make a good impression, but I got so much out of it anyway. I'm not certain I was the right type for the female dancers, and I was going to work plenty in the next few years. I also kept Bobbie Bates and Stan Mazin as friends for years to come. I went to Egypt twice with Stan in our senior years as he became an Egyptian tour guide, post dancing. I was obsessed with Egypt.

In 2000, I also went back down to Carol's *The Carol Burnett Show 33 Year Reunion* in Studio 33, that Stan got me invited to, and actually got to meet Carol, as I had not before. She is such a gracious, lovely lady. Ken Berry was there too, and I got to talk to him. He didn't remember me from 1974, but this was now the year 2000.

CHAPTER SEVENTEEN

THE BRADY BUNCH VARIETY HOUR, A NON-CHAPTER

So, dear readers, this is the only full TV series I did, all thirteen shows over a three-month time period. It also has a very interesting, beautifully illustrated companion book that was published in 2008, titled *Love to Love You Bradys, the Bizarre Story of the Brady Bunch Variety Hour*, written and produced by Lisa Sutton, my friend Ted Nichelson, and *Brady Bunch* cast member Susan Olson, who was Cindy Brady on the series.

I was a supporting cast member, along with seven other swimmer/dancers, yes, swimmer dancers, as we did dance and sketch routines with the Bradys, but also what is now known in the Olympics as Artistic Swimming, a competitive sport. We were not nearly as skilled as the teams are now, and almost like the 'cavewomen' of the sport. We were better than the swimmers in Esther Williams movies who were held up by men and wires, but just not as advanced as today, as we learned how to do the sport in six weeks and did a new routine a week. The teams that compete in the Olympics and other world titles work for months on a routine, and practice for hours a day. We were called the *Krofftettes,* as Sid and Marty Krofft were our producers.

I highly encourage the reading of this wonderful book, as there are many celebrities who guest-starred in the show and many stories about them, and I have a lot of stories in it that I relayed to Ted in numerous interviews. It's much more thorough than I could put in this book. Try looking for it at your public library and it is still for sale online as well. Do give it a look-see!

CHAPTER EIGHTEEN

HERE COME THE STARS

Al, being the Rock Star, had other Rock Star friends, and actors he knew. Whenever we went to a concert together, we almost always had backstage passes or free tickets. Back in '75, Al had to do a session and wasn't able to go see the Rolling Stones, but knowing how I loved them, sent me with our friend, graphic designer and photographer Gary Nickamen.

It was the Star Stage Tour, where the stage unfolded like a star, and Mick Jagger had a cherry picker to ride in, above the crowd. Gary was this very hilarious Jewish fellow who looked like a walrus—short of stature, with a huge moustache and beard and semi bald head. He was completely safe for me to hang out and laugh with. (I loved laughing and still do.)

We did NOT have backstage passes as Al knew I had an eternal crush on Mick Jagger, so he wasn't going to do that without him being there. The Stones knew Al from him playing with them on "You Can't Always Get What You Want." Gary and I had free tickets in the Stones VIP section that was up and to the right of Star stage. Two seats in front of us were Ryan and Tatum O'Neal who conversed a lot but seemed to be getting along. In front of them was Elizabeth Taylor.

The show, however, was a sloppy and rather disappointing event, with their music all over the place and a stoned Mick Jagger rolling down the star points of the stage. Some of his singing wasn't that good and was off pitch, but Gary and I sang along with a lot of the songs, to make up for it.

Al and I went to see Leo Sayer at the Troubadour for free, as Doug Westin and Al were friends. The Troubadour had a great bar, and we hung out there with Glen Fry of the Eagles before the show, as Al and he were friends.

I excused myself to use the ladies' room, and when I returned, Glen had gone to his seat, and we went to ours in the balcony to watch Leo's show. Al told me that Glen told him that I was the best-looking woman in Hollywood. That was a huge compliment from Glen, as he was dating the Playboy Playmate of the Month at that time. Leo's show and music was fantastic! He was still singing "Up on a Tightwire" in whiteface like a clown, and it was very special.

We went to see Linda Ronstadt and the Eagles at an open-air arena somewhere in L.A. County a few weeks later and hung out with Linda before her set. Al said, "Linda, meet Linda," a nice icebreaker, and she was sooooo down to earth for being a major singing star.

We sat at a picnic table backstage. It so happened that Linda was living in Atlanta for a while, at the same time

Al was. She thanked Al for turning her onto an outlet store that sold fashionable, cheap jeans, really just talking about everyday stuff. I was surprised that she looked more average than her pictures and album covers, with little makeup on.

We found out later that we shared the same physician, Dr. Cantor of Beverly Hills. He'd give her eye drops for her photo shoots that enlarge the iris, that make your eyes look bigger. Her eyes always looked huge on her album covers, and that explained why.

The Eagles went on first, and we had seats in the second row, and of course their music was great, but they sat on stools and were so boring to watch. Sorry, I like some movement.

Then Linda came on and she also just stood in the middle of the stage, and now she was just wearing a plain everyday dress, instead of her cute cub scout shirt and shorts and dancing more, and once again I found it rather boring even though she was a fantastic talent.

The next concert we went to see was the Spinners at the Greek Theater and that was great. Al's best platonic female friend was Julia Negron, wife of Three Dog Night frontman, Chuck Negron. Julia was very self-confident and fancied herself a Rock and Roll QUEEN as she had a lot of gossip and Al loved the gossip. He liked gossip more than I did, especially about his competition, their wives or girlfriends, what kind of money they were making, with what manager, what drugs and drug problems they had, that sort of thing.

We picked her up in the limo, (we took waaaaay too many limos), and the three of us had great seats close to the front of this marvelous open-air venue, that had more of an intimate feel than the Hollywood Bowl. I'd danced to Spinner's music for the last three or four years and really got down to their music. The lead singer came down from the stage and danced through the aisles and I stood and danced along with him. It was my kind of concert.

After that, Al got us tickets to see Elton John. We did not go backstage but had wonderful free seats. This was when Elton did all his costume changes, did handstands on his piano bench, the big sunglasses, etc.

Next, we got free tickets to see David Bowie at Universal Amphitheater, yet another great open-air venue. It was Bowie's Diamond Dogs Tour, with his two black Diamond Dogs dancers that he held on long leashes as they leaped and boogied at the ends of their tethers in front of him. He was in his thin white Duke persona and dressed so classy and looked so handsome. I would've loved to go backstage, but Al didn't know him, so we did not. He was definitely one of my "British Invasion" favorites, and a lively performer.

We went to see a band called Pages at the Troubadour, but this time the frontman/leader of the band, Richard Page, was an alumnus of mine so I had the connection. Al really loved this band, and Richard Page was Danny Zuko to my Patty Simcox in the production of *Grease* I did at SPA. He was a sweet blonde guy who was a talented singer and musician. We went backstage after the show and Al was happy to meet him.

He wanted to work with him, but I don't think he ever did. About seven years later, Richard formed a new band called Mister Mister and had a huge hit called "Broken Wings."

Al took me to the Roxy on Sunset, just up the street from The Whiskey, but he would not tell me who we were seeing. The Roxy was an intimate club like The Whiskey, but on the whole had better acts and clientele.

We sat at a table and ordered drinks and Al said, "You'll like this, but I won't, so enjoy." A sort-of balding but attractive man came and sat down at a baby grand piano on the stage and played amazing songs that were more dance songs. He got up and danced and played the maracas while his drummer played solo. His name was Peter Allen, and he was fucking wonderful! He played "I Go to Rio" and in the middle once again got up and danced and played maracas. He was also married to Liza Minnelli for a while, but he was bi and contracted AIDS and died only a few short years later, way too soon.

Al was a huge Steve Martin fan, and Steve was doing his standup comedy act at The Roxy in the early days of his success, when he wore his white suit, did the arrow-through-the-head thing, and balloon tricks. Al didn't know Steve but worshipped him as much as Lenny Bruce and was determined to meet him.

Al called the editor of *Crawdaddy*, a music publication, and told them he wanted to interview Steve for their magazine, and somehow John Belushi was added to the mix. I wasn't working and I was hanging out at the pool when a photographer from *Crawdaddy* arrived with a white background screen and lighting and camera equipment. Then Steve and John arrived together.

Al interviewed Steve first and offered them both lemonade, and Steve asked if we had any chips. I did find some Frito's in a bag, but we didn't eat chips, so I don't even know how they got there. I put them in a bowl and Steve kept walking around looking at our house. When I finally gave him the bowl and Steve took some, he said, "These chips are stale Linda," but was nice about it.

I apologized but I had no others and realized I needed to keep snacks around. At least John and Steve liked the lemonade. Then it was time for the picture to accompany the interview for the magazine. The three of them stood in front of the screen and did Steve's "wild and crazy guy" finger point, and after a couple of shots, Al had me join them in my bikini behind him, and that's what made the magazine. I was referred to as a "foxy friend." It was an iconic picture for me. Before they left, Steve took Al aside and asked about the "foxy friend" but alas, I was taken. I guess Maureen McCormick and I were his type.

So now there is a steady stream of Al's musicians and celebrity friends coming to the house. My friends are welcome as well, but they're not famous. Most of the time, if not all the time, it was with very little advance notice. I was busy as well, auditioning or working, so there really wasn't a lot for them to do most of the time except maybe have a beverage and hang out for an hour or two.

Jay Ferguson, the singer for the band Spirit, and his gorgeous girlfriend came up one afternoon for the usual beverage, and they were so beautiful, with movie star good looks. I was a big Spirit fan, so I was starstruck and tongue-tied. They didn't stay long and after they left Al told me he thought they might've been interested in a four-way. I thought to myself, "How does he know this?" but I said nothing. That was, once again, not me.

One Saturday, Al invited Alice Cooper up to watch the game on our big screen TV in the living room. Alice arrived after the football game had started with an entourage: Bernie Taupin and his wife Sheryl, who was also a professional dancer, and a bodyguard. The bodyguard carried a medium-sized cooler with beer in it and Sheryl carried a small cooler with Jack Daniels in it. Wow, they had their own beverages!!!

Bernie and Alice were also rather wasted-looking from those beverages, but not Sheryl. It was about two in the afternoon, and I thought that Alice and Bernie made sort of an unusual pair of friends, but opposites do attract. Alice had the most stunning blue eyes I'd ever seen. Sheryl was sweet and sooooo young to be married. We talked a little and found out that we were both dancers. Sometime later, we saw each other in Joe Tremaine's dance class every once in a while, or at auditions. We both got chosen to do a summer replacement show on *The Captain and Tenille,* but neither of us did it. Thank God! The production routines I saw were just lousy and sloppy, the worst I'd ever seen on national TV.

Anyway, Al showed them around the house, and they sat down and had a beverage, but they didn't seem to be that interested in football, as they looked like they were going to fall asleep. They left shortly after that. A few years later Alice did get clean and sober with the help of a strong faith and his loving wife Sheryl, and they are still together, married, and Alice is still a force of nature rocker and performer at 76!

One Sunday morning Al gets a phone call and tells me that his actor friend Peter Riegert and his girlfriend Bette Midler would be coming up to spend the afternoon with us. OMG and OH FUCK! BETTE MIDLER! She has been one of my iconic singers and actresses since college, and of course I still sing "Boogie Woogie Bugle Boy" in Ray's show.

It's not even noon yet when they arrive, and Bette is petite and rather quiet, and Peter is young and innocent looking. We ask them what they'd like to drink, and they both say coffee, so I start up my Mr. Coffee, as I drink that every morning. Bette says she wants half and half in hers and I put some in, but it curdles and I'm so embarrassed (I only used sugar at that time), but she drank it anyway, as it's all I had.

We go out to the pool and hang out in shorts and tank tops. We have some hot dogs that Al makes for all of us, and I bring out some mustard and mayonnaise to put on them but I'm the only one to put both on mine. Bette and Peter think that's so funny and call me a shiksa for using the mayonnaise. They all think that's funny because the three of them are Jewish, mustard only, but I get a kick out of it too.

Then Bette wants to go and read a magazine she's brought with her, so she goes into the "balling ally" for about an hour and I leave her alone. Peter, Al and I went and hung out by the pool some more and then they split but I could hardly talk to her. I had a problem back then with being starstruck. They did tell me that they found it refreshing that I barely wore any makeup, as all of the other dancers they knew wore a lot all the time. I hardly wore any when I wasn't working, I mean why? I had good skin, and who wanted false eye lashes at home.

The next time we saw them they came up and brought food from Nate 'n' Al's deli which was delicious. Bette had very little of her corned beef on rye sandwich but Al, Peter and I wolfed down ours. Bette was on the "liquid protein diet" that was all the rage, and she had lost weight, but I told her to be careful. I could put my fingers around her wrist it was so tiny. That was the last time I saw them, and I still didn't talk to Bette very much, boring for her, I'm sure, memorable for me.

Next up to the house was Carly Simon and Danny Kortchmar and his then-wife. Danny was a session guitarist and also guitarist for James Taylor, although James Taylor wasn't with them. They were in town from NYC and staying at the Beverly Hills Hotel.

As I understood it, Carly and Mrs. Kortchmar were good friends, and Danny was penning a song that James would release in 1977, "Honey Don't Leave L.A," my favorite James Taylor tune. They toured the house and then they invited us down to their bungalow at the hotel for a late afternoon tea. We got more dressed up than the usual bikini and shorts we usually hung out in and headed down.

If you've never seen the bungalows at the Beverly Hills Hotel, they are a wonderful place to stay, at the back of the main hotel, elegant but cozy, and everything is decorated in pink and green. It's very tropical, like the Royal Hawaiian in Hawaii.

It was just the five of us, and tea consisted of mostly wine and weed. I never smoked weed much in public, I didn't smoke weed much at all, as it made me paranoid AND stupid, but I did enjoy some Pouilly Fuisse white wine, although I usually never drank in the daytime.

After about an hour or so, I felt no pain, but it was time to go. On my way out the door I bent down and gave Carly a kiss on her big, beautiful lips, and she didn't seem to mind. It was a bold drunken move on my part but unforgettable for me. The only time I saw Carly after that was walking with her two kids in Central Park when I was living in NYC in 1982, after my Broadway show closed. I didn't say anything to her. I did know that she was living at the Dakota, where John Lennon had been living when he got shot.

Now my friends DID come and visit me, my showbiz friends and friends from my hometown of Bremerton. Some came down to check out the Hollywood scene thinking that "If Linda can do showbiz, so can I." Not so much, not without the proper training, and putting money into your career i.e. professional headshots, resumés that were typeset, and of course, a place to live. Hundreds if not thousands of young people try the Hollywood scene if not for movies and TV, for the music industry as well, year after year. But for most, it was a quick in and out and back to Bremerton, or wherever they came from. Except one.

I hung out with teenage boys from East High School as they were nice to me AND they had good musical taste. One that I had a crush on but never really went on a date with, had me over to listen to all the latest bands and smoke weed in his basement bedroom as both his parents worked. I would do so on occasion, when I wasn't in dance class. His BFF was a guy named Kevin Eddie, who was a star basketball player at East High, a hilarious, Harlem Globetrotter-style basket baller whose games I'd go see just to watch HIM. He was an outgoing, charming personality with a Rod Stewart pineapple hairdo, always looking for a good time. I'd hang out with the two of them, and they were the darned cutest teenage boys in Bremerton. I felt very fortunate.

One day I got a call, and it's from Kevin. I invite him over to the house the next day and he tells me his story, as I hadn't seen or heard from him in five years. He didn't want to go to college, so he did some bartending work, and then went up to do labor on the Alaska pipeline for about three years.

He saved his money, bought a cute sports car, and drove it down to L.A. and got himself an apartment, all on his own. He had decided he wanted to be involved with the music industry as a recording engineer and had been going to every major recording studio in L.A., handing out resumés with no luck whatsoever. I was proud of him that up until a day ago, he hadn't called me looking for a helping hand knowing that I was with a record producer. But after hearing his story, I was bound and determined to get Al to help him. Al came home from whatever he was doing, and I fixed the three of us something everyone could eat, and I could tell Al liked him. I think I should mention that Kevin also dressed like Robin Williams at that time, with striped T-shirts and suspenders on his jeans and looked like Rod or Robin, as well, I mean he had it going on.

So, here's what Al came up with. He had his shelves of records surrounding the white baby grand in the alcove, and when Al wanted to listen to one, he'd just put the record back in its jacket and gently toss it to the floor behind the piano on the thick shag carpet and they formed a big messy pile for weeks at a time. They were in alphabetical order, but Al was too rushed and too lazy to put them back. So, if Kevin would come up once a week for the next month and put the records in order on the shelves, he'd help get him a job at the Record Plant as a janitor, as that is how you started in the recording industry, like starting in the mailroom of a corporation, ya dig? Dropping off resumés would get you nowhere, so are you in, Kevin?

"Oh, hell yes," was his quick reply, and we were all happy for the opportunity. I believe Al knew that Kevin would fit into the music industry like hand in glove with his looks and "Wild and Crazy" Steve Martinesque personality.

Kevin fulfilled his verbal contract to Al, and dutifully came up to the house once a week and put the records away and Al worked his magic and got Kevin a janitor job working for the Record Plant, and then in no time he became an assistant engineer which was one step up from janitor, moving speakers and equipment when the bands and artists came into the studios to record. They are supposed to be watching and listening to the engineer and the producer as much as possible to learn the board. It was fairly complex with numerous channels, tracks, and volume levels to adjust. But that never quite happened.

Kevin was almost too popular and fun for his own good with some of the male stars at the studio, in particular, Rod Stewart, Ron Wood, and Paul Stanley of Kiss, and a pretty boy band called Angel that basically went nowhere— they were just pretty boys.

I'm sure there were a few others, but these are the ones I remember him telling Al and me about. He played basketball outside in the back lot with them, but he also partied with them. Cocaine was the drug of choice, and lots of it. So, instead of learning the recording board, Kevin became their gofer for their wants and needs.

I saw less and less of Kevin, and he'd also got an apartment with the other assistant engineer in the heart of Hollywood, and they were a cute party duo, too much so.

I'd ask Al from time to time, when was doing some work there, if he'd seen Kevin and he said that sometimes he'd see Kevin's big red nose coming around a corner in a hallway of the studio.

Then one day, Kevin called us complaining that one of the Rock Stars, the one who was notorious for his drug use, was calling him and waking him up at 3am looking for drugs and wanting Kevin to go and get some for him!

That was quite frustrating for me and Al because we had high hopes for my friend, but at this point his plans were being derailed by the partying and drugs. We both told him to take his phone off the hook and just start distancing himself from the men doing that to him.

But alas that didn't work, and we grew apart from him as we were both working a lot, and we did not do any blow or weed. We did smoke cigarettes but controlled even those (two a day for me), and drank some wine, but no hard liquor. We wanted to work.

I heard that in 1980 Kevin had gone back to NYC to work with John Lennon on a new project, and he was there when John Lennon got gunned down. It upset him so much that he quit trying to be an engineer and moved back to where his father lived in Yuma, Arizona. He went back to bartending and lived a more peaceful existence, until his passing 30 years later at 60. People from our hometown still think of him as a Rock Star, but most never knew of his unfortunate experience with a precarious industry—ooh baby baby it's a wild world.

CHAPTER NINETEEN

CARS, CARS, CARS

To say that Al bought too many new luxury automobiles is an understatement, and people told me it's what led to his financial problems later. Yes, he'd gotten rid of the Rolls and the Maserati and yes, he'd purchased a Cadillac, and a Mercedes, but those were just not flashy enough for his taste.

Shortly after we were all moved into Freebird Mansion, he purchased a 1976 Excalibur Phaeton two-door fire engine red with a convertible hood. They were modeled off the 1928 Mercedes-Benz SSK, and quite the focus pull. Rod Stewart, who I saw one night going to an acting class, was driving around L.A. in his, with the convertible top down and a scarf flying from his neck. Al liked to drive with the top down too, sans scarf.

One day when I came home from work, I went home to a closed garage and Al came out to our parking lot to greet me. He then opened the electric garage door and inside beside the Excalibur was a 1974 Jaguar XKE model in forest green with a black convertible hood ... FOR ME?! MY OH MY!

Now I had not asked for a new or different car at all. I was fine driving the Corvette, but the engine was so rough from being neglected, it was sort of disturbing to listen to. So, we got in but before we went for a ride, I had to warm it up for about five minutes to get the engine ready to drive, a must. But frankly, my dears, both cars were not me, both just too much car for me, heavy cars with a lot of horsepower, and I'd heard that Jaguars were problematic machines over the years.

I thanked him of course, and he went to the Jaguar dealership and traded in the 'vette for me. About ten days later I had a rehearsal at UCLA, as I was taking an extension class from one of my previous acting teachers from SPA, the British actor Charles Vernon.

I was doing a scene study class on a weeknight but meeting my scene partner at the school in preparation for that, on a Sunday, mid-morning. I had moved the Jag out to our little three space parking lot next to Al's two other cars and started the car to warm up, per my instructions on its use. I went back inside the house to gather my script and purse only to see the Jaguar on fire. YIKES! I turned it off, but the fire continued and thank God Al was home with me!

He got on the phone and called the fire department who did arrive quickly, but they had to drive up the hill to our cul de sac that we shared with our one set of neighbors to the right of us. There were about eight homes on either side of Dalegrove Drive, staggered below us, and many of the neighbors, especially their kids, came running behind the firetruck that of course had its siren going.

They put the fire out quickly, but there sat my beautiful British mode of transportation looking very destroyed, and it was. We discussed if I had done ANYTHING differently than just turned the car on, and I did not. Al got on the horn to the Jaguar dealership owner in Beverly Hills, and he came up for a look-see and to take the Jaguar back. It was fairly clear from where the fire had burned that it was inside the cab, not the engine.

So, after the research was done at the dealership it was discovered that the seat belt was incorrectly attached to the controls at the dashboard and caused an electrical short. I hadn't even touched the seat belt that morning as I had never gotten that far. I'd sat down once to start the engine only and left.

I drove the Cadillac for a while, and Al did get a full refund from the dealership. I looked at a couple of different styles of autos, as Al still wanted me to have a car. The two I was interested in were a two-door 1957 T-bird, turquoise blue with portholes in the roof, and the new Datsun 280Z.

I auditioned a lot and did grocery shopping, errands, etc., so it was decided that the best choice was the 280Z. The T-bird's engine was original and too fragile—I needed a workhorse car. So, I got the favorite car of my life at that time, a copper-colored 1976 280Z, two-door that lasted me for 11 YEARS! It was $7,000, as was the Jaguar—that's what cars cost back in the good old days.

Around this time, Al also informed me that his only son, Brian Kooper, lived with his mom, Al's first wife Judy and her second husband, an attorney, in Laguna Niguel, about an hour south of us. I knew Al had a son, but I thought they lived back in New York where he was born. I was shocked and dismayed that Al was not connecting with him, and I was going to change that. I told Al to get on the phone to his ex, Judy, and arrange for him to come and visit for a weekend, and soon. In a couple of weekends, Al went down to Laguna Niguel and got Brian, who was 11.

He was a nice young boy who still had a lot of kid left in him, and we had plenty for a young kid to do: our dog Bozo, the swimming pool, the pinball machine, and hot dogs and hamburgers.

Al took him down to the Record Plant to show him where he worked and show him off. Then I took him home strapped into my new 280Z, and we sang Beatle songs together, and this happened again on a semi-regular basis. I also really liked his lovely mother with her kind demeanor and beautiful almond eyes. Al and his son Brian are still fairly close to this day. I am happy it worked out for them.

I was still working a lot for Sid and Marty Krofft after *The Brady Bunch Variety Hour* folded after one season. I did a TV special for one of their Saturday morning kid shows that featured a cute prefab group called Kaptain Kool and the Kongs that starred Michael Lembeck as Kaptain Kool. Some of the Krofftettes agreed to dance for them if we had a featured singing and dancing routine. But instead of letting us sing, they hired three other female singers who could do impressions of celebrity singers and one who played drums. We got a dance where we played cowbells and had some attractive closeups, but once again, a job's a job.

Later that summer, my girlfriends and I did another job for the Kroffts, performing a great opening dance routine for a TV special introducing Sid and Marty's latest nighttime venture called *The Krofft Comedy Hour.* Our production dance routine was very challenging, the hardest Joe Cassini, the Krofft choreographer, had ever created for us. I was given a solo with a prop whip, then was joined by all my other girlfriends for the ending.

Al was working too, producing more artists, this time for Epic Records. Al had heard that Epic had signed Ricky Nelson and Al had wanted to produce an album for him for a long time. They told Al okay, but first we want you to produce a new artist named Marshall Chapman who was a South Carolina rocker, a 6-foot-tall woman who came with her own band and songs that were not very good. But Al was getting paid for it and he did the best he could with her.

Then, as promised, he got to produce Rick. Rick was doing a residence contract at the Aladdin Hotel showroom in Vegas. One of my best girlfriends and roommates from SPA, Denise Esola had bought a house in the 'burbs in Vegas and had been dancing for the Tropicana and MGM Grand shows. I wanted to see her, so Al invited me for the weekend. We got a room at the Aladdin, and then I went to see Denise for the day, came back to the hotel, changed into a dress and went up to meet Rick in his suite with Al before we went to see his show. An assistant let us in, and we went into the sitting room of the suite where Rick was sitting in a chair.

When he saw me, he stood up (and I could tell it was for me) and he extended his hand and shook mine. Then he said hi to AI and told us to have a seat which we did. It was a beautifully decorated hotel suite, and Rick was a soft spoken, handsome man.

We stayed for about fifteen minutes and then excused ourselves to get a bite to eat, and he looked at me and stood again. Ozzie and Harriet had taught him such gracious manners! We told Rick we'd see him after his show. His Stone Canyon Band was very enjoyable, playing many of Rick's old hits from the 50s.

The next day at 11am, I spent about fifteen minutes by the pool watching my skin turn darker shades of brown in front of my eyes, but it was too much, too hot, approximately 115-degrees, and I went back up to the room. My first experience with Vegas heat.

I left Al and Vegas, took an early evening flight back to L.A. while Al was going to stay in Vegas and work with Rick on his choice of songs for the album, all of which were covers of wonderful pop songs from good writers, my favorite being "Chump Change Romeo" written by Danny Kortchmar.

When the album was finished Al played it for me in its entirety, and it was EXTREMELY enjoyable. We were both so excited for its release. Al took the finished product to Lenny Petze, the man in charge at Epic, and he told Al it was the worst piece of shit he'd ever heard and it would never be released.

It was shocking to hear that, as well as hurtful, and Rick had no power over this asshole. In a few short months Rick was killed in a private plane crash—so young, so heartbreaking. Al again approached Epic and suggested that it be released in Rick's honor and again was told to "Fuck off, it's never coming out, we still hate it!"

At least Al got paid and at least I got to meet Rick Nelson who I'd grown up with on TV, but just another of life's many disappointments of being in the music industry.

During this period of time, I was really trying not to take as many dance jobs and focused on getting more acting jobs with my dear agent Bill.

The agents seemed to want to put you up for the "BIG SCORE" starring or co-starring roles at that time, and I felt he should've just started me off with under-fives on TV series and the like, but it seemed to fall on deaf ears. I was put up for parts against Donna Mills, Goldie Hawn, and Sally Field, already big stars, and me with almost no film credits, just dancing/singing credits and a one-liner (thanks Bruce Kimmel) in *The First Nudie Musical*, and on a McDonald's commercial.

I was sent on an audition for *Smokey and the Bandit 2* for the part of Burt Reynold's girlfriend, and the casting director told me right off the bat "I'll let you read for this Linda, but Sally Fields has the role, she's Burt Reynolds' main squeeze." Well, duh!

I then went and auditioned for Renée Valente at Columbia Pictures for soaps, and I was offered a job acting on a soap, but I turned them down for oh so many reasons. I mean if you wanted a steady job, you had one, and they've always liked good looking men and women, but you are a slave to them, you live, eat and breathe the character day and night and have like one day off a week. Every night you go home, eat, clean up, memorize lines, and go to bed. Wash. Rinse. repeat. I just didn't love acting that much. I loved Al, my pets, my home, and my friends.

The one thing I should've done, and I encourage any young film actor to do, is take a cold reading class. That would've helped me so very much. You HAVE to take a commercial acting class, that is necessary for TV commercial auditions and camera technique. I ended up teaching commercial acting for almost twenty years. I'm retired now and loving it.

After the disappointing album incident with Rick Nelson, Al was ready to put out a solo album for himself, as he hadn't done so in four years. Stan Polly, Al's agent, and I were all for it! At least it would get released.

Al sort of did what he did for Rick Nelson by picking some songs from other writers that he could relate to that were semi-pop, and then about another five that were his own. He wrote "This Diamond Ring," for Gary Lewis and the Playboys in the 60s but now he made it funkified and a lot more enjoyable. Plus, he wrote a song for me "Turn My Head Towards Home," very loving and romantic, and another at the end of the album called "Hollywood Vampire," about an episode of *Night Gallery,* starring the ethereal Lesley Ann Warren as a vampire.

Al was famous for his album covers when he had artistic control. They were so eclectic, and creative and included *Child is Father to the Man*, which was his idea for the Blood, Sweat & Tears album, *I Stand Alone*, his first solo album with him as the Statue of Liberty, and one with his second wife Joan, *New York City, You're a Woman*. Now he decided his next album would feature both of us on the cover.

There was a famous picture of Jane Fonda in Life Magazine from the 60s, nude on the beach—so artfully done, covering her breasts and crotch with strategically placed arms and legs.

He hired our dear Norman Seeff to shoot us in studio separately, in the Jane Fonda pose, and then transferred our heads onto one another's bodies. He named the album *Act Like Nothing's Wrong*, which he got from Stevie Wonder's touring road crew's T-shirts, get it? The inside sleeve photo was inspired by a photo of Arthur Miller and Marilyn Monroe, when they were together. Hugging and looking like Al is my great protecter, his idea also, and I did love it.

I love the whole album—soft forlorn love songs and poppy songs and good horn and string arrangements. I took the cover to the best print agent in town, and it started my print model career. Her name was Joan Mangum and she's still my friend and alive to this day. She's a very enjoyable woman, pretty herself, and it was a joy doing print work and print jobs for her. It is fun to go out and shoot for an hour or two and not have to exert myself physically or mentally that much, just listen to directions from the photographer, and do the facial expression and hold still. My hourly rate was $110 an hour and $650 day rate.

My favorite print job was going to Santa Barbara to shoot a brochure for the new Ford cars coming out in '77. It was me and a very pretty black model just going from location to location in stunning Santa Barbara, in different outfits, standing by the cars, looking pretty and happy.

The photographer and his assistant drove all of us up in his van, with all our clothes, and from location to location. Then, after about two hours, it was time to eat! We went to about three restaurants and had great seafood meals, fresh from the Pacific Ocean. I got along nicely with my lovely fellow model, and we discussed music.

My model friend found out that I loved Parliament-Funkadelic (or P-Funk). She was going to his concert in a couple of weeks back in L.A. and would I like to join her? WOW, and hell YES! She gave me her phone number and told me to call her a couple of days after we got back so we could make plans.

When I got home that was the first thing I told Al about, not the $650 day gig. "I'm going to go see George Clinton and P-Funk with my new African American model girlfriend, and I wants to get funked up," I joyfully exclaimed!

"Oh no you are not," Al firmly replied, "it's just a little too ethnic for you." This is coming from a man who loved black people, R&B, had lots of black musician friends, but he felt overwhelmed if outnumbered. He was absolutely NOT racist. So, I didn't call her and never saw her again, and no "Mothership Connection" for me.

Al decided he needed to tour his new album and pull a band together to do so. He found a married couple, who I found kind of eccentric, and a drummer, so it was just the four of them, no horns.

They'd start off on the East Coast and would make their way across the country in the Fall and Winter of 1976. I was trying to get more acting roles, so I was auditioning a lot, plus, I was trying to stay in town as much as possible so Al could travel more if needed. He was the big moneymaker compared to my gigs.

We looked at his schedule and it was decided that I would join him in Boston for Thanksgiving week, but before that, I'd get to visit my 90-year-old great grandma Iva in North Carolina. I'd never met her, just been around her as an infant.

I flew into Atlanta airport as it was a hub for Carolina and got fogged in. I slept on my suitcase overnight, and they did get me to Asheville, North Carolina the next day. My great aunt Lou "Lulu" Cassaro drove into Asheville to fetch me and take me to my grannie's tiny house in the tiny town of Silva, North Carolina. My grannie lived in a 600 square foot "Dollhouse". I believe she was the oldest person I'd ever met at that point in my life. She was pretty wrinkled, and she had big boney hands, and was thin. She had a small dowager's hump, and she did not talk much but she smiled and looked happy. I slept upstairs with my aunt in a loft bedroom with a mattress on the floor. We had to climb a skinny attic-like staircase to get there.

The next day was Thanksgiving and the three of us went to Denny's somewhere between Silva and Asheville in the breathtaking Great Smokey Mountains, a treat for me. It was a good traditional meal with turkey and all the fixn's, and then we went back to the doll house where some of my hillbilly relatives were coming over to meet me. We all shared the one bottle of champagne I had brought with me, which was very sweet.

The next day I'd be flying to Boston to be with my love, as I had to get back to L.A. to the house and pets. I was so glad I got to do this even though it was short, and I'll never forget my grannie's hugs, with her large, boney hands. She was able to live in the doll house for the next four years alone (the neighbors kept an eye on her) until her passing at 94. It was the only time I visited her.

I need to mention that I got a call at my grannie's house from my agent Bill Meiklejohn. As fate would have it, it was pilot season, and I'd been chosen for a TV pilot. I'd been auditioning like crazy and getting more relaxed and focused with my auditions. This audition was for an understudy role on a new live action *Archie* comic book series. I'd read for Betty and for whatever reason, after they'd chosen her, the casting director and director thought I was the better choice. So, I was called to come back to L.A. and come into rehearsals as understudy to Betty, and then if it went to network, I'd replace the actress they'd chosen as Betty.

This call came in the day I got to Silva, and I had spent next to no time with my grannie. I mulled over the request for about five seconds and apologized to dear Bill, but I told him I was seeing my 90-year-old great grandmother for the first and possibly only time, and I just needed to stay for HER. But, if it did go to network, I'd be on board to replace the Betty character. My dear agent understood my dilemma.

The Archie pilot premiered a couple of months later and it got a horrible review in *Variety*, and my agent was told it was a no go for the network. Thankfully, I didn't miss anything by not doing it.

I was so happy to see Al. I hadn't seen him in about three weeks and had missed him so much! We had sex of course, as I was only staying for one more day. Then we had dinner, and then the band rehearsed.

The band was also rehearsing the next day, so I took myself sightseeing on the historic yellow brick trail in downtown Boston. It was a line of yellow bricks that led to statues and small museums in historic Boston. It had begun to snow lightly and was pretty and romantic for my final night in Boston. Al would be opening in Boston in about three days, but I needed to get home. The band that would be opening for Al, traveling from East to West across the U.S., was a new band called Tom Petty and the Heartbreakers, and I would see them when they got to L.A.

I had also re-enrolled in college as an undergrad at USC as a full-blown acting major, but I was only going part time, one class per semester. I had enough college credits from the other two schools to give me Senior status, so I thought "why not?" I could do it slowly as it was expensive, but I'd saved enough money to pay for it myself.

My next audition was an interesting one. Bill called me and said, "You've got a 'go see' for a new movie, *Ode to Billy Joe.* It's for the principal role of Billy Joe's teenage girlfriend, Bobbie Sue. Are you familiar with the song by Bobbie Gentry?" "Very much so," was my reply. He said, "Here's the deal though. Max, the director, wants you to go to his house, and you probably won't get to read, it's just an initial and true look-see for type. The Max is Max Baer, do you know who he is? Jethro from *The Beverly Hillbillies*, and he's a director and producer now."

"I'd read about it," I replied.

"Good," Bill said, and he gave me the address, blah blah blah, and appointment time.

The address was in Beverly Hills, off one of the Canyons, a big, beautiful home. I was nervous as I'd heard many stories about Max. He was quite the womanizer and at that time had a porn star girlfriend that was very provocative for the '70s.

But I got in my Z and went. When I got out, he was outside with a table set up on his porch and an assistant there. Jethro was a tall, muscular man, 6'4", nice-looking, just like on TV. He spoke in a normal manner, not the hick accent and energy I was used to. He had chairs at the table and thanked me for coming and asked me to take a seat.

I gave him my headshot and resumé. He looked at it, asked me a couple of questions, and said, "Well, today is just preliminary, and we'll let Bill know," and then I left, no sexual harassment, very professional.

I did not win the role, Glynnis O'Conner got it, and did a great job. Frankly she was a better type than me for the role, and the movie turned out to be a huge success.

AUDITIONING! Somebody could write an entire book on that alone, maybe they have? I don't know, it'd be a horror story, I'm sure. I had several well-trained and educated actors tell me they simply could not endure a career in entertainment because auditioning was too stressful, the acting, dancing, singing, any of it. It was also an on-going, never-ending process, that was few and far between, unless you became a HUGE star and then the industry came to you.

For every ten auditions, it has been researched that you'll get about one job. You spend more time driving to and from auditions than working. It also required getting dressed, hair and makeup, and studying any script they may have given you ahead of time. If you are fortunate enough to get that script ahead of time, DO MEMORIZE IT, even if you need to hold it in one hand, which you can do, but never in both hands.

Most auditions are in a public rented space, not some private home, apartment or hotel room, where you can run the risk of being harassed or even raped. There is usually an element of nervousness, as it's a job interview, a job that you need, to pay rent, buy food, or support your family. It's your income! There were a handful of times when I was just called or told you've got the job if you want it, and those were totally gold.

Finally, the casting directors were kind, and they generally never told you then and there how you did. The only rude casting people I ever encountered was in Seattle, where I later moved and taught acting. These were non-union jobs, and the casting people could get away with being cruel.

Al was winding his way across the country from Boston with his band and Tom Petty opening for him. It was about a month before he landed in L.A. Due to the booking contracts, Tom Petty and the Heartbreakers would be coming in before him and playing their own gig at the Whiskey and Al would be arriving a few days after that and playing solo at the Roxy.

Al insisted that I go to the Whiskey before he came back to see Tom Petty open for Blondie, fronted by Debby Harry herself. He'd make sure a friend of mine and I were comped at the door. I took a male rocker friend of mine from USC, and we sat at a booth at the back of the club. It simply amazed me at the lack of people there that night. Nobody had heard of Tom Petty and the Heartbreakers yet, but Blondie was fairly well known. The club held about 300 people and there were only about 50 in the house.

Tom and his Heartbreakers hit the stage, with two more guitarists and a drummer behind them, so it was just a quartet. I tried like crazy to get a handle on their music, as it seemed kind of Pop/Rock. The three musicians, with Tom in the middle, were all dressed in black, head-to-toe, not unusual, but they were all so thin that I found it distracting, and the black made them look even thinner. I felt the name of their band should've been "The Rocking Malnourished," as all I could think of was somebody should get those boys to eat more, but they were gifted musicians.

The Heartbreakers left the stage, I hoped to go get a hearty snack, and Blondie and band came on. I was much more familiar with their songs, and I did enjoy their set except that Debby Harry was thin and had a large head and wide face, so she looked like an orange with popsicle sticks for arms and legs. It was a challenging night for me visually, but we made it through to the end.

Al came home two days later with another three days before he played the Roxy. He told me immediately that that night we'd be on a double date with Tom Petty and his girlfriend to see *Richard Pryor in Concert* at the Shubert Theater in Century City.

Now Al was crazy about comedians Lenny Bruce, Steve Martin, and Richard Pryor in particular. I had only seen Steve Martin live at the Roxy after he'd come to our house for the *Crawdaddy* interview he'd done with Al. His show was not that different than what I'd seen him do on TV, doing stupid balloon tricks, and was a fairly clean show with few F bombs. I was in for a big surprise with Richard Pryor.

We met Tom and his girlfriend outside the theatre, and it was nice to meet him. I told him I enjoyed his show, as I didn't go backstage at the Whiskey. He was sweet and kind of quiet, as was his lady. The three of us were in our early to mid-20s, Al was 32, and, as it turned out, the dirty old man.

We went in and found our seats and I sat next to Tom, with Al on my right, and Tom's date to the left of him. Etta James opened the show and then came Richard Pryor, and close to two full hours of him. Richard's jokes just got dirtier and dirtier, and Tom, his girlfriend, and I, sunk further down into our seats and when I glanced at them they were blushing at much of his material, and I'm sure I was too.

Meanwhile, Al was laughing his ass off, clearly not embarrassed by any of it, having the time of his life. I have as salty a sense of humor as anyone, as anyone who knows me will tell you, but YOWZA, tough trade even for me.

After the show, we said goodbye to Tom and his girlfriend, and I never saw Tom again, in concert or socially, other than film of Tom in concert in his later years.

He'd become such a commanding presence on stage, I was quite proud of his development as a frontman. I wish I would've been able to see him just one more time and say, "Remember the time you double-dated with me and Mr. Kooper, and we saw Richard Pryor?" I'm sure we'd have had a giggle! He left us too soon, eight years ago as of this writing, from an accidental prescription drug overdose. It was such a loss, and I was honored to have double-dated with him.

Al had only one concert booked for one night in L.A. It was sold out and since the Roxy had festival seating, we had several hundred of our friends there in a crush outside the door jockeying to get in for a good seat. It was a good show. His band was tight, and my boyfriend looked great, although it is kind of a blur to me now.

That was his last show promoting the record, the tour ended, and the band went to other jobs elsewhere. Al had had some issues with club owners along the way on the tour and he was burned out. The album had mediocre sales at about 40,000 copies, but it did get a *Billboard Magazine* award for a promotional advertisement in 1976.

CHAPTER TWENTY

I "MONKEED" AROUND

Spring came early in L.A. We really didn't have much of a winter in Southern California, as it rarely got below 60-degrees, except maybe in the months of November to mid-February.

It is now March, with lovely weather, and my birthday month. My girlfriend Coleen had been doing some modeling for Playboy, appearing in their storyline pictorials that were artistic and not at all sleazy. She had a natural, womanly figure, nothing artificial or augmented. Some of you may remember the issue featuring womens' bodies with bird heads on them. My friend did that! It was very classy, and beautiful. She was now getting invited to Hef's Friday night parties with a lot of celebrities, many of them male and somewhat older, in their 40s and 50s. Hef also had Sunday evening parties, but those were quieter, and not as star-studded.

She invited me to come with her as a sort of birthday gift, but it was not ON my birthday, it was the Friday before or after that. We got dressed up and took her car, since she knew the way.

Al wanted to come, but she could only take one guest, and only single young women, which was the strict rule. It was obvious why that was when we arrived. We drove into Holmby Hills, even more exclusive than Beverly Hills, to a road with a private driveway and gate. To the left of the driveway, going up a small hill, was a large rock, with a speaker on it, about four feet high. There was a buzzer in the rock, and someone would answer and ask your name. If you weren't on the list, you could not get in. When the gate opened, we drove up the short hill and there it was, on the left of the circular driveway, the famed Playboy Mansion. There were two valets who took your car, gave you a claim ticket, and the car disappeared to a huge lot out of sight.

We approached the giant carved dark wood doors, and a door butler let us in. We entered a spacious high-ceilinged foyer with a bar straight ahead, dining room to the right, and a movie theater room to the left. There was also a winding red carpeted stairway to the left that went to the second floor.

We went to the bar and got ourselves a glass of wine, then we went into the dining room to find a place to sit. We were fortunate enough to find a small table for two. There were about three long tables and some smaller ones that seated three or four. We recognized many celebrities dining and conversing, including Ryan O'Neal, Dennis Cole, Tony Curtis, Kareem Abdul Jabar, a very thin Clint Eastwood, and Barbie Benton with a group of Playmates at a table of their own.

I also recognized John Raitt and his wife, who I would say hello to later, as I'd done *Camelot* with him at Music Circus. We set our wine and purses down and went to the steaming buffet to choose and plate our dinners. It was good wholesome American cuisine, well cooked and fresh, nothing exotic.

I noticed Hugh Marston Hefner walking around, shmoozing with different people at the tables, with his pipe, silk pajamas and satin bathrobe, looking very happy. As I started to eat, I looked across the dining room, and looking right back at me was Mickey Dolenz of The Monkees. We held each other's gaze for a long thirty seconds and then I took my gaze away and continued to eat and talk to Coleen.

We finished our dinner, and I went over to John Raitt to say hi. He didn't remember me, since it had been almost four years earlier, but he was nice to me. We then stepped outdoors to have our after-dinner smokes. We also had another glass of vino and went out to look at the pool area and backyard. We couldn't see the atrium or monkeys, as it was now dark.

We went back inside and discovered it was movie night, as that is what happened on Friday nights, with Hef sitting with Barbie, front and center, and many rows of seats behind them for everyone else.

The movie did not interest either of us, so Coleen suggested we put on bikinis kept in a locker dressing room and go swimming in the grotto pool instead. The bikinis were hanging on a rack, clean, and in different sizes. There were lockers with keys to store your clothes and purses—so impressive!

The grotto was very provocative and magical with its low ceiling made of hewn rock and rockery on the sides of the pool with low lighting and steam that rose from the heated pool. It was just like I'd seen in photos in *Playboy*, that I had looked at from time to time. We got into the lovely, heated water and then, and out of the blue, here comes Mickey Dolenz in swim trunks to join us.

He says, "Hi ladies," but his eyes are on me, not both Coleen and me. He heads on over to me and sort of gently pushes me away from Coleen to the far end, towards the side and shallow end of the pool, saying nothing. Then he gets behind me and pulls my bikini bottoms down, and he takes me from behind, with no foreplay necessary, as we have lots of moisture. He goes fairly fast and furious—it was over in about two or three minutes—he pulls out and lifts my bikini bottom back up to my ass. What a gentleman! If this isn't a "zipless fuck" I don't know what is? Huh, Erica Jong?

So, the three of us just hung out, not really swimming, just relaxing and sipping wine for a few minutes, saying next to nothing. I excuse myself because I have to pee, and Collen tells me there is a half bath where we came from, so I get out and go into it. I didn't have time to lock it before the door opened, and guess who's there? Yup, that Monkee Mickey wanting more, wow!

He pulls my bikini bottom off this time, and we go again, again from behind, fast and furious and erotic as hell for me! He finishes, says something like, "See ya later," and exits the bathroom. I guess he was done "Monkeeing" around.

I go back to the pool and Coleen is ready to get out now. We go back to the dressing room that has showers, take a quick rinse off, get dressed and head home, out the back end of the mansion, as the entrance and exit are one way. She just smiles at me with a knowing smile, but we don't say much about the encounter, and it was all good.

A couple of weeks later, I went to Emerson-Lowe Photography for an interim head shot, as I'd made the mistake of cutting my beautiful long hair to shoulder length, and needed a current one until I could grow it back.

Who do I see at the other end of the large photo studio? ALL the Monkees doing some new shots, as they were touring now. I take a seat to wait for Sam Emerson, Tony Lowe's partner, to come and talk to me, and Mickey runs over with a shit-eating grin on his face. He says, "Hi, how are you today? You sure look good!" and I say, "Oh I'm fine, but I have a boyfriend who is friends with Sam & Tony, so be cool".

He got it and went back to the other band members. The Monkees had to change their clothes, and Sam put me in front of his lights, shot about a dozen frames, and I exited quickly.

Was I guilty of cheating on Al? Not at all because we never talked about ME being physical with other men now, did we? It was not revenge sex, it was a one-time fling, and I'd heard from various sources that Al had done what he said he'd do and had some one-time sexual encounters with groupies. This was my one and only time in almost three years that I had done so, and I planned to keep it like that, if I could.

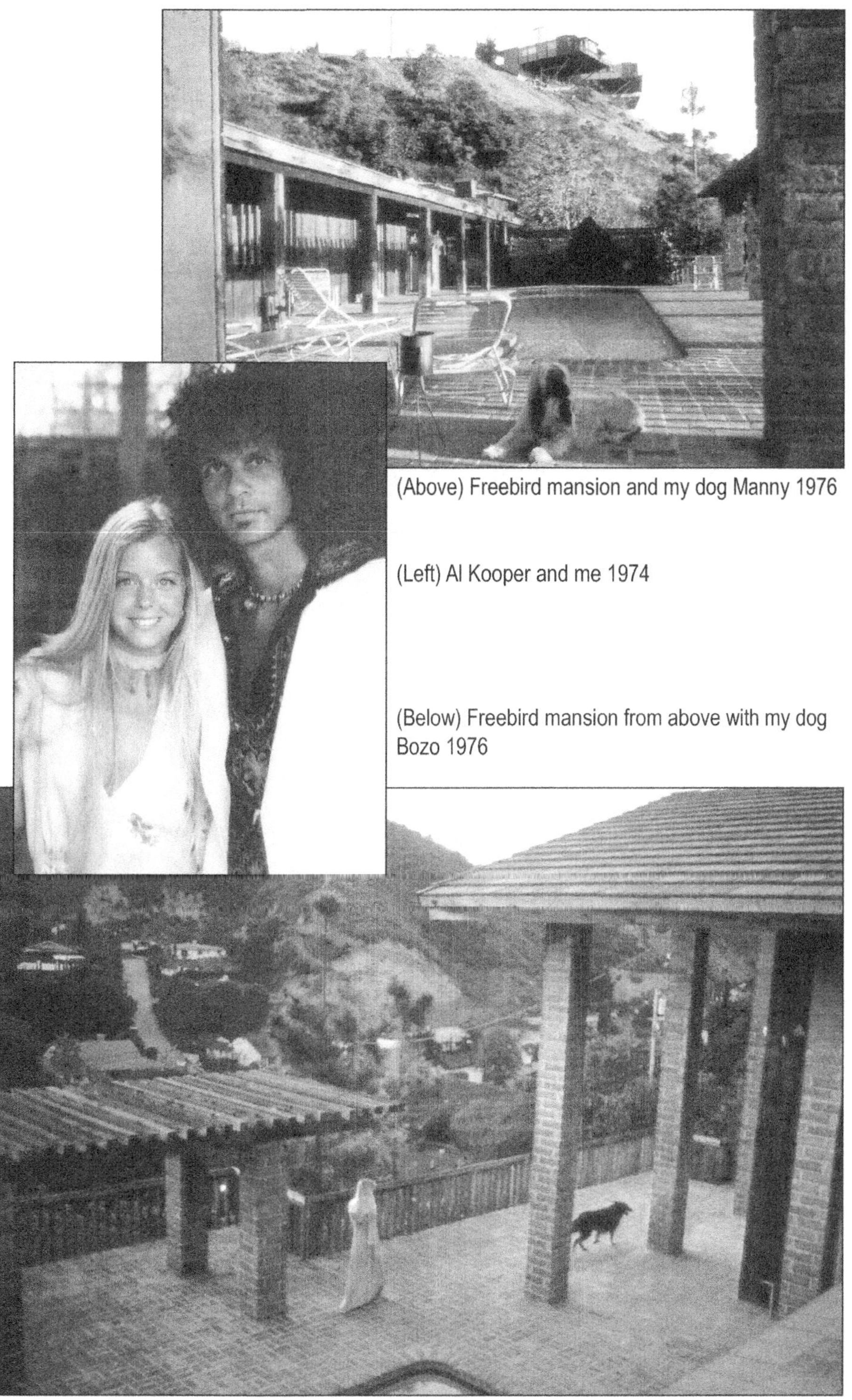

(Above) Freebird mansion and my dog Manny 1976

(Left) Al Kooper and me 1974

(Below) Freebird mansion from above with my dog Bozo 1976

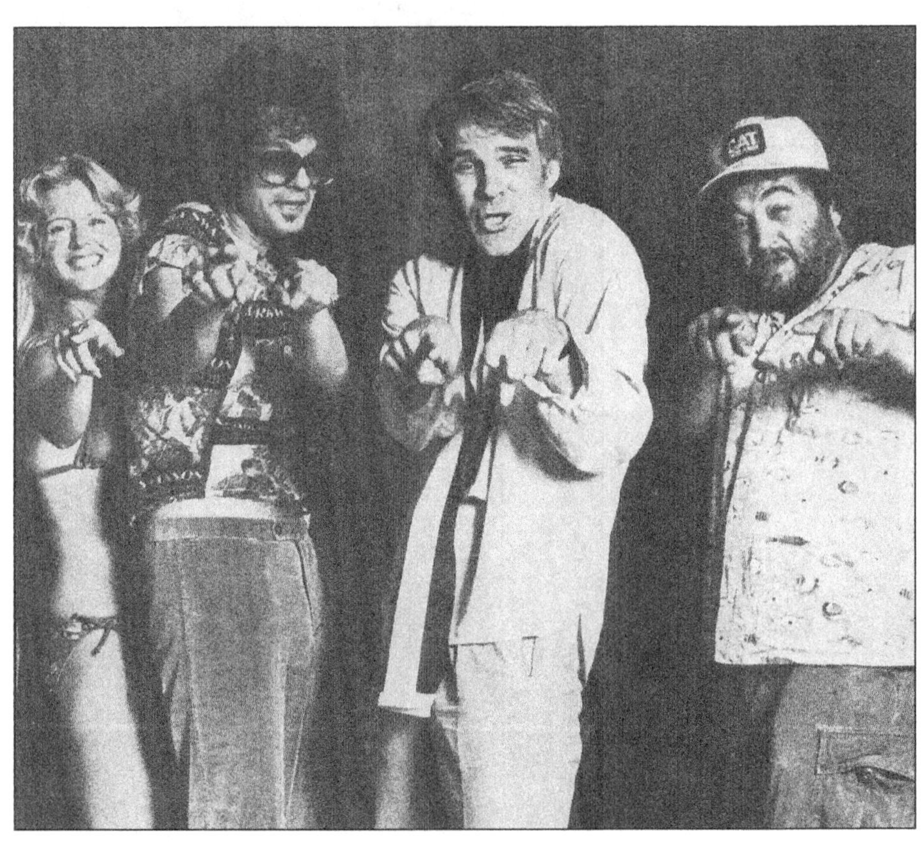

Me and Al Kooper, with Steve Martin and John Belushi, who visited Freebird mansion for an interview with Al.
I was invited to join them for a PR photo.

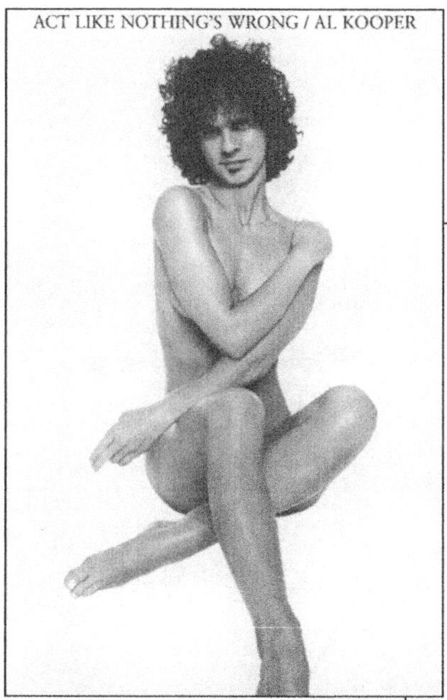

(Above)"Act Like Nothing's Wrong,"
front album cover,
United Artists Records, 1976

(Right) "Act Like Nothing's Wrong,"
back album cover,
United Artists Records, 1976

(Below) "Act Like Nothing's Wrong,"
inside album sleeve,
United Artists Records, 1976

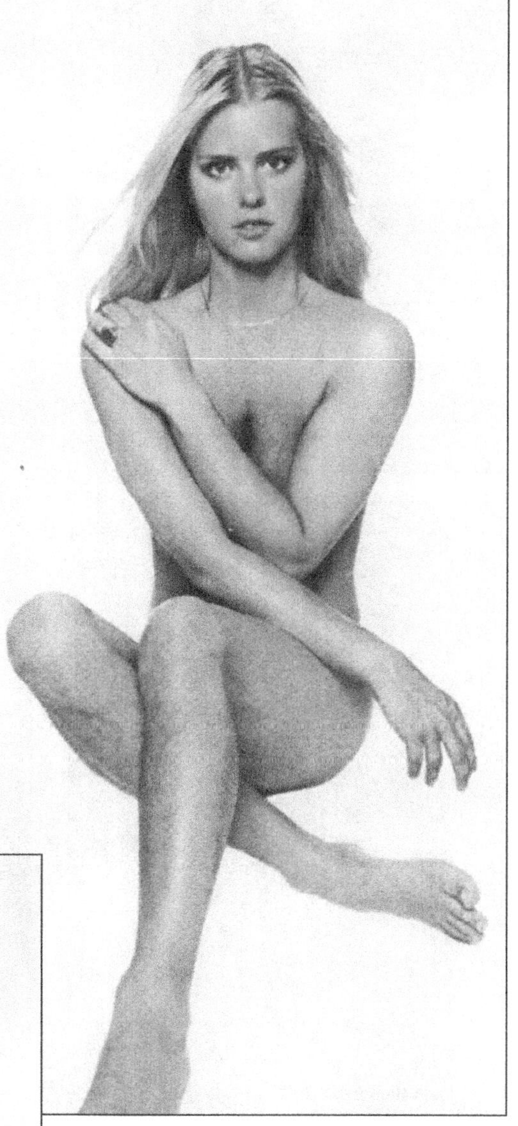

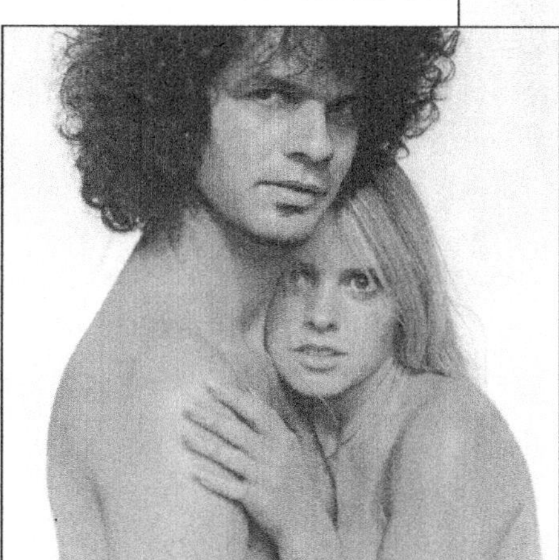

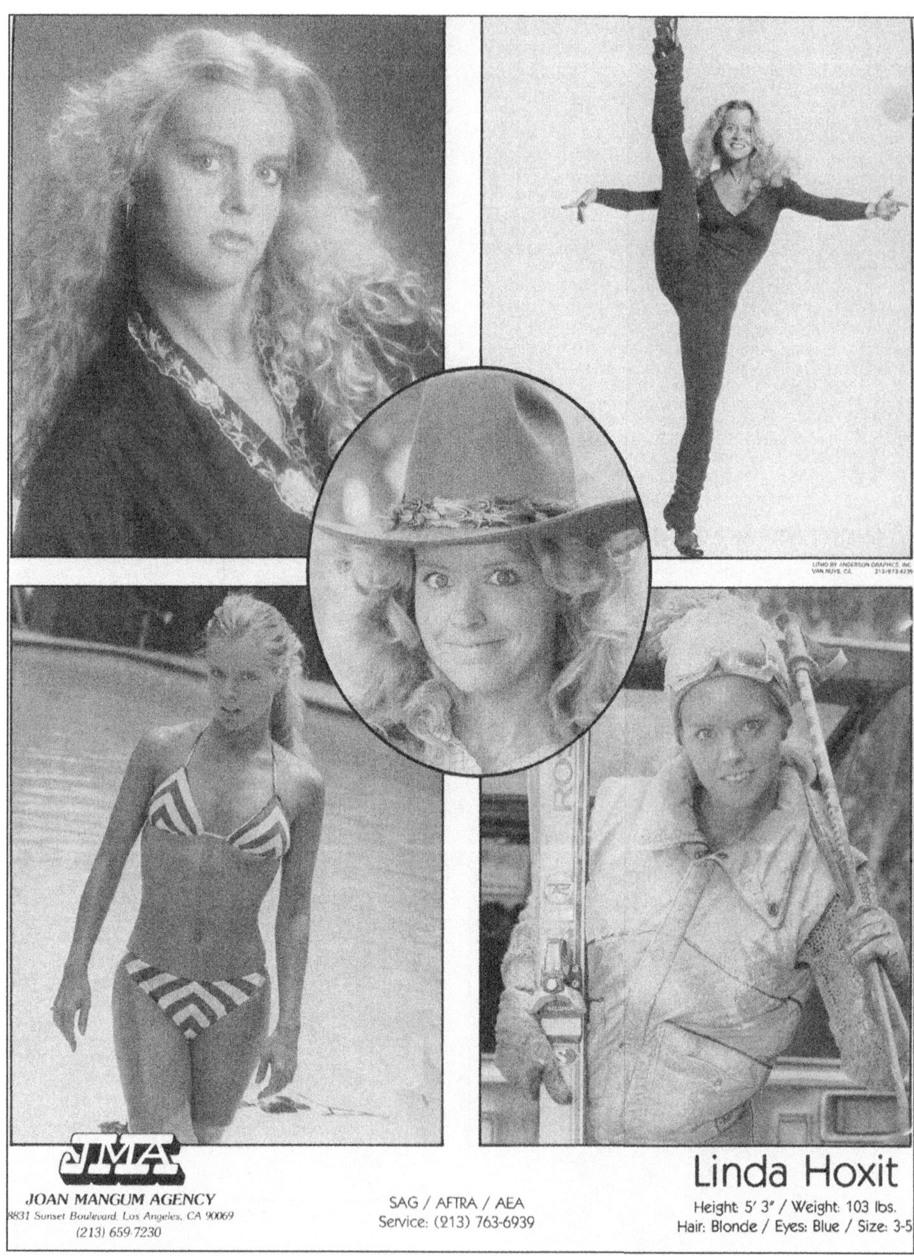

(Above) My ZED card, JMA Models and Commercials Unlimited

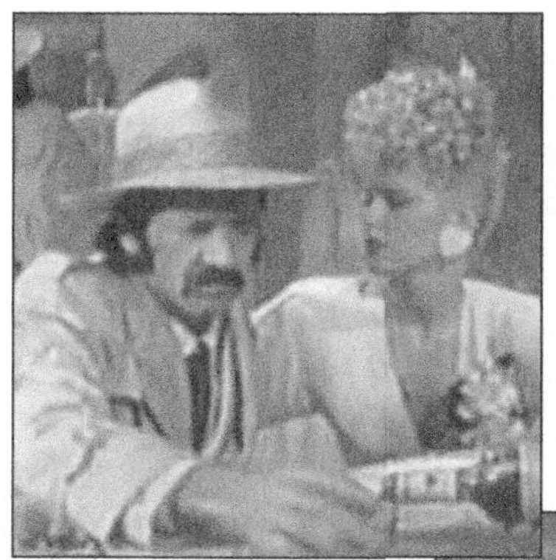

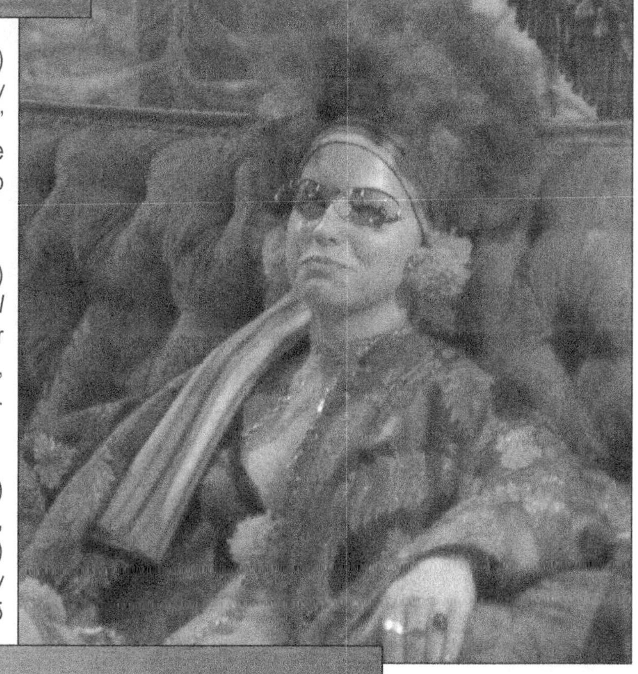

(Above)
The Sonny and Cher Show
"Case of the Missing Case"
acting scene
with Sonny Bono

(Right)
The First Nudie Musical
as a sex worker
at Wanda's Brothel,
and my first screen line.

(Below)
As a drum majorette,
(I'm at the far right)
The Smothers Brothers Show
1975

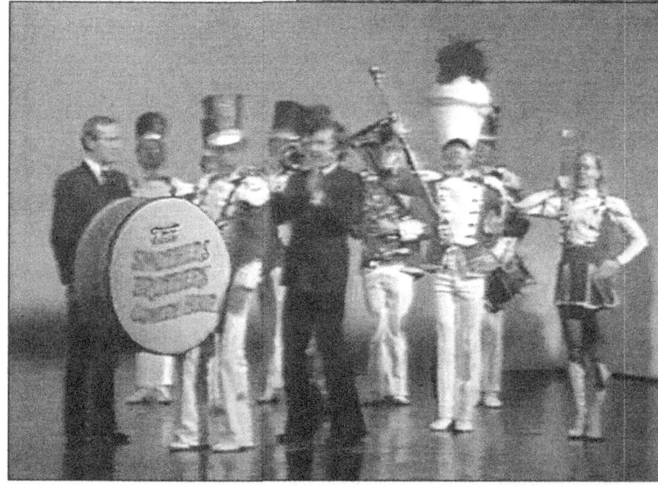

The photos on this page are screen captures and the quality is not as sharp as I would like, but I wanted them included because they're so iconic.

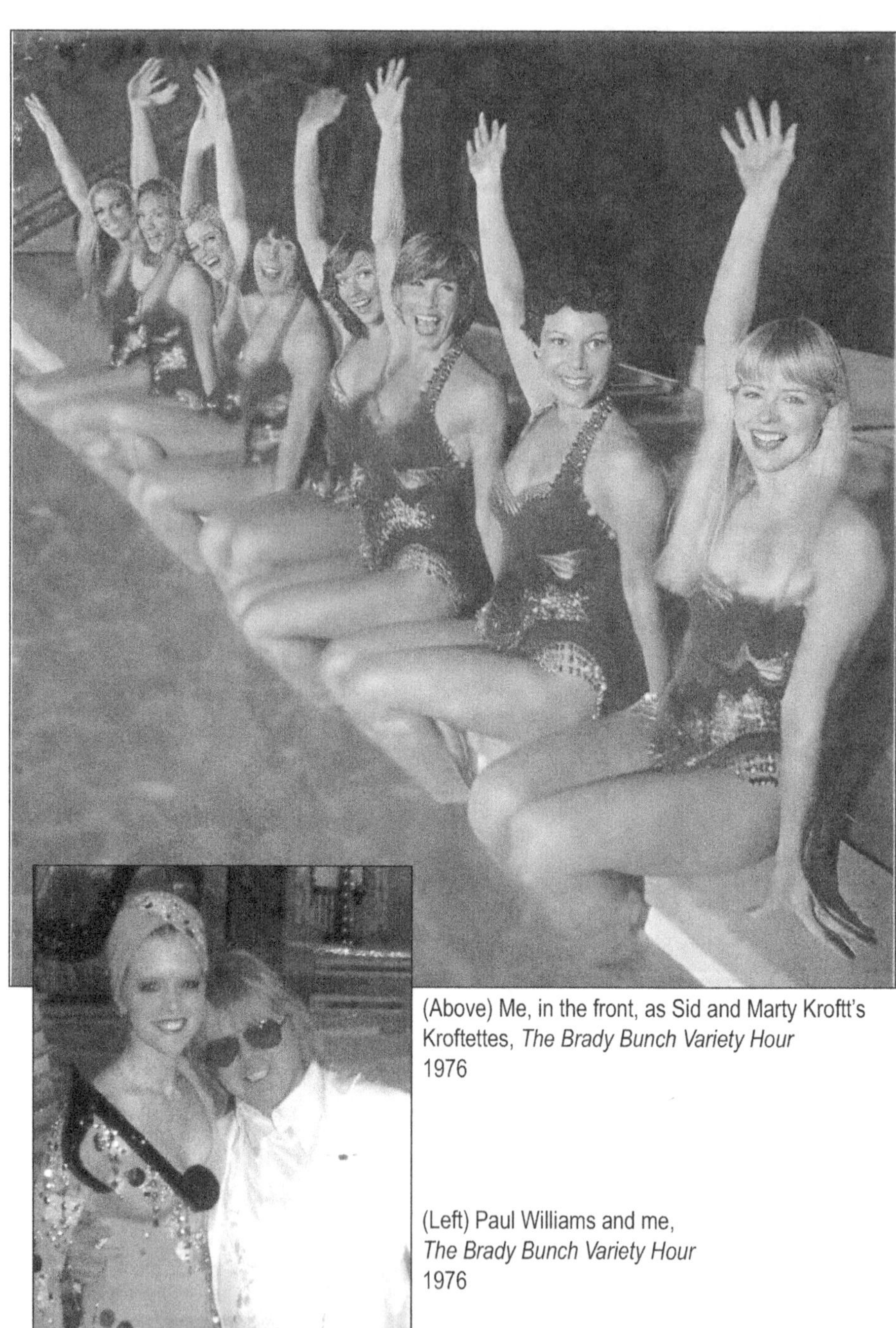

(Above) Me, in the front, as Sid and Marty Kroftt's Kroftettes, *The Brady Bunch Variety Hour*
1976

(Left) Paul Williams and me,
The Brady Bunch Variety Hour
1976

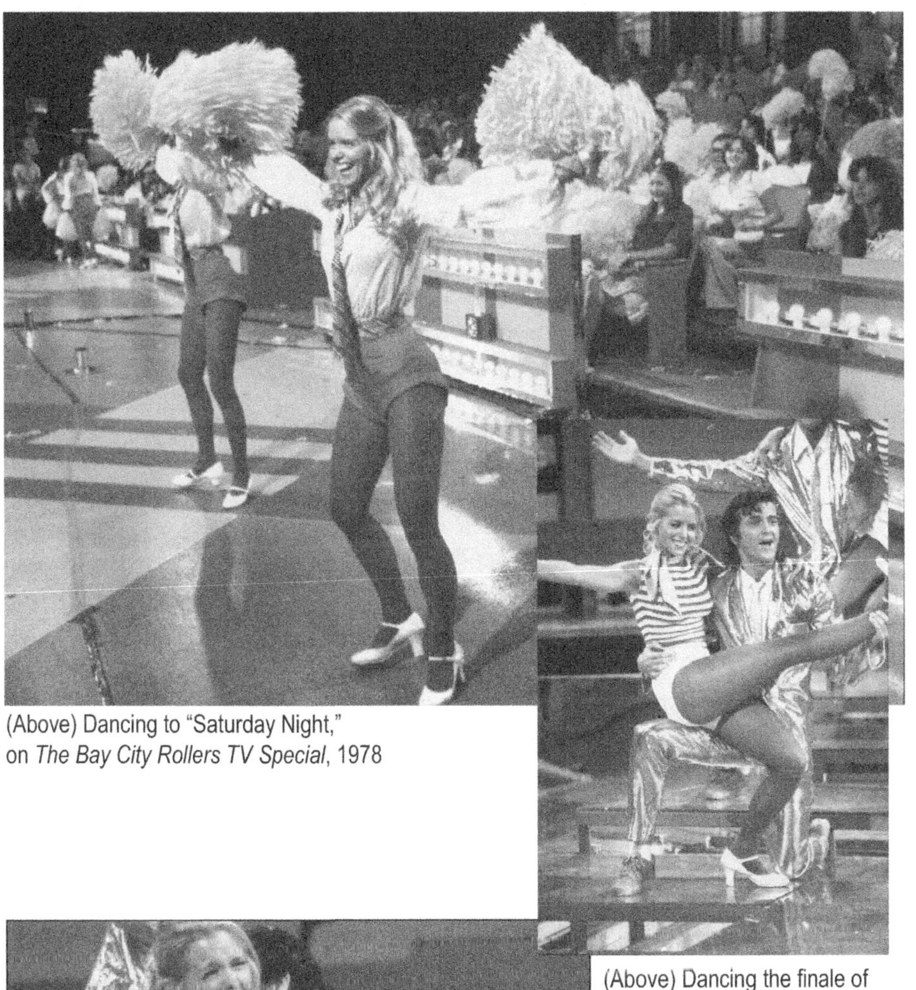

(Above) Dancing to "Saturday Night,"
on *The Bay City Rollers TV Special*, 1978

(Above) Dancing the finale of
The Bay City Rollers TV Special,
with Leslie McKeown, 1978

(Left) Leslie McKeown biting my neck on the *Bay City Rollers TV Special*. He became my new boyfriend the next day.

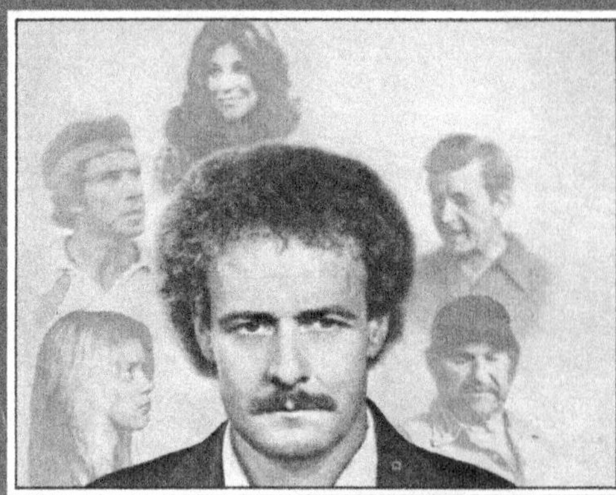

If Jesus came in the 20th century, how would we respond to him?

Join **THE INVESTIGATION** and find out!

A powerful new motion picture about the cost of Christian discipleship—and the glory!

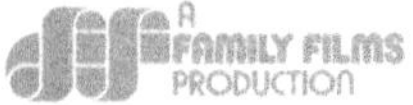

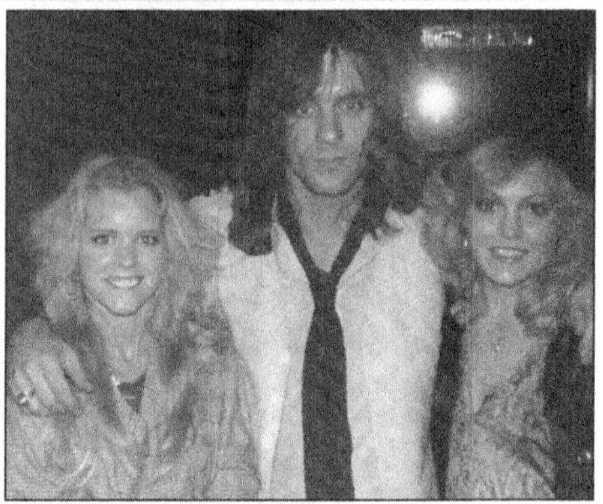

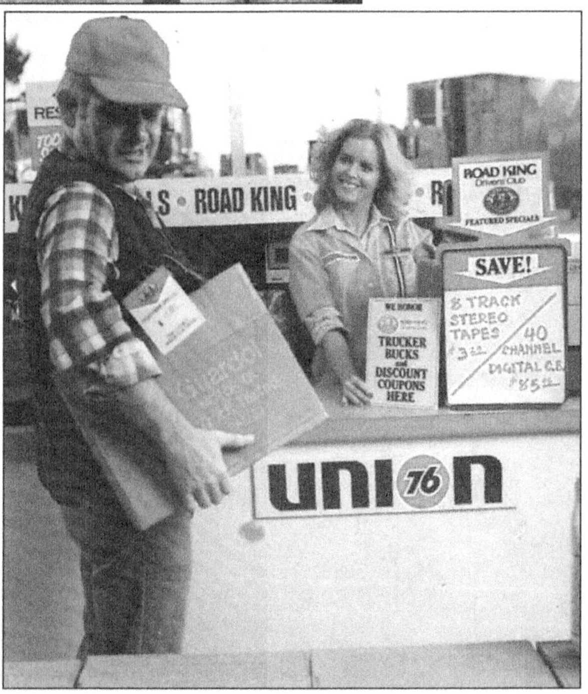

(Top) The religious film, *The Investigation*, PR poster. I am bottom left as a modern-day, reformed Mary Magdalene.

(Center) BFF Bridget Johnston and me filming the HBO TV Special, "Opening Night" with rock star Eddy Money. 1979

(Right) Modeling print job for Union 76 1980

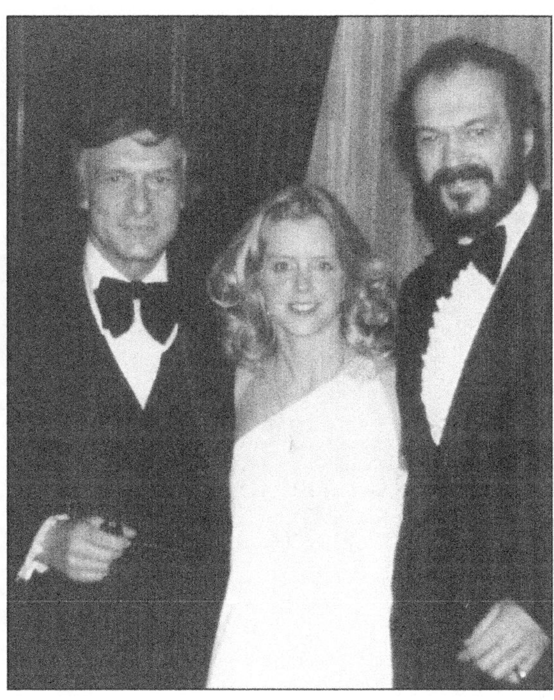

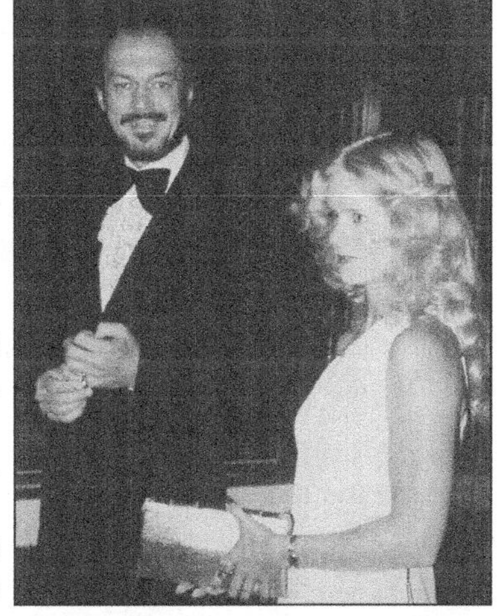

(Above) Hef, Keith, and me at the Playboy mansion tribute event for Frank Sinatra.

(Right) Keith and me at the Frank Sinatra event.

(Below) Keith, Hef, and me going to the Playboy Jazz Festival 1980

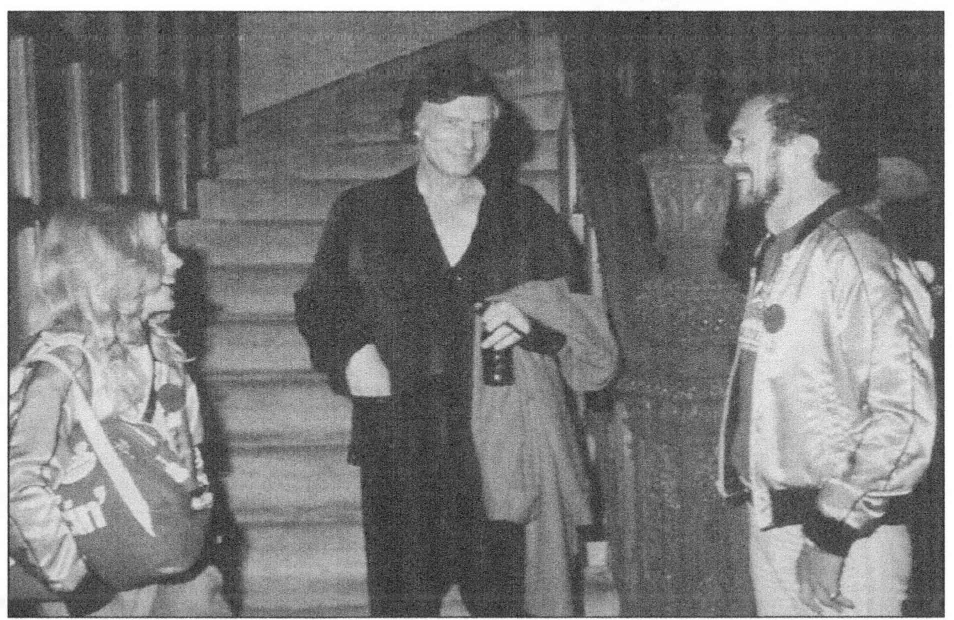

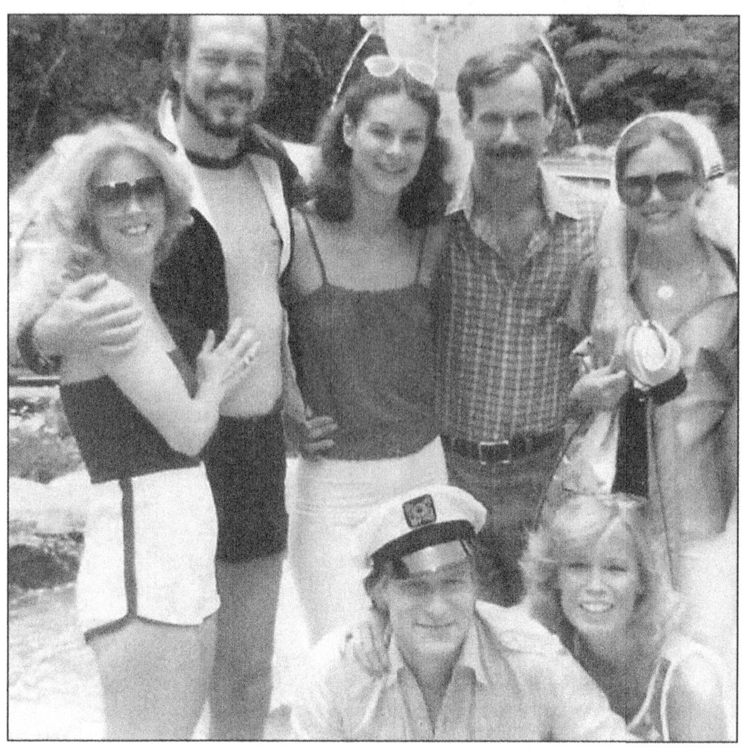

(Above) Sailing Day with the Hefner family. Keith and me, Sondra and Hef, Christie Hefner and David Gunn, Johnny Dante, and date. 1980

(Below) On the sailboat; Top, me as the "the crew", left to right, Sondra and Hef, Christie Hefner and David Gunn, Johnny Dante and date.

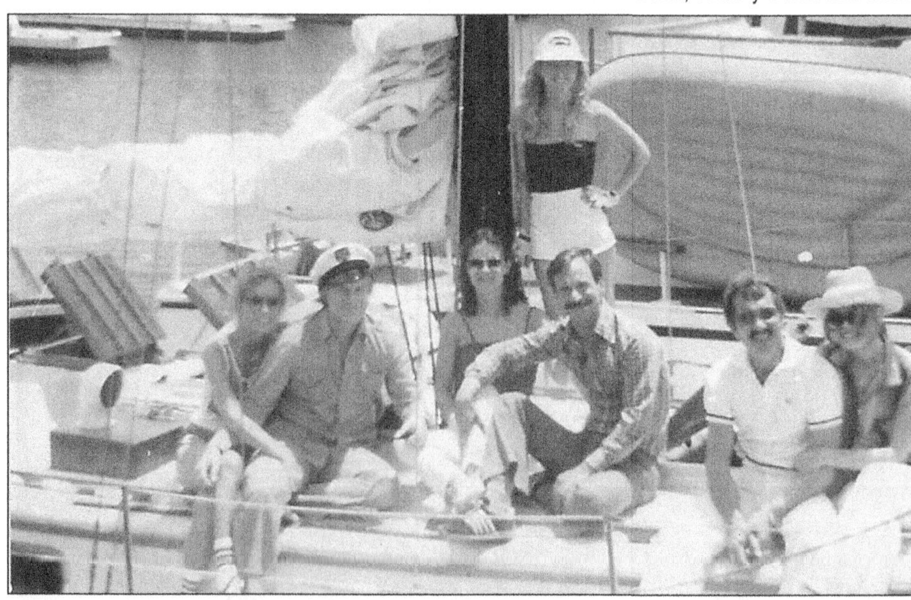

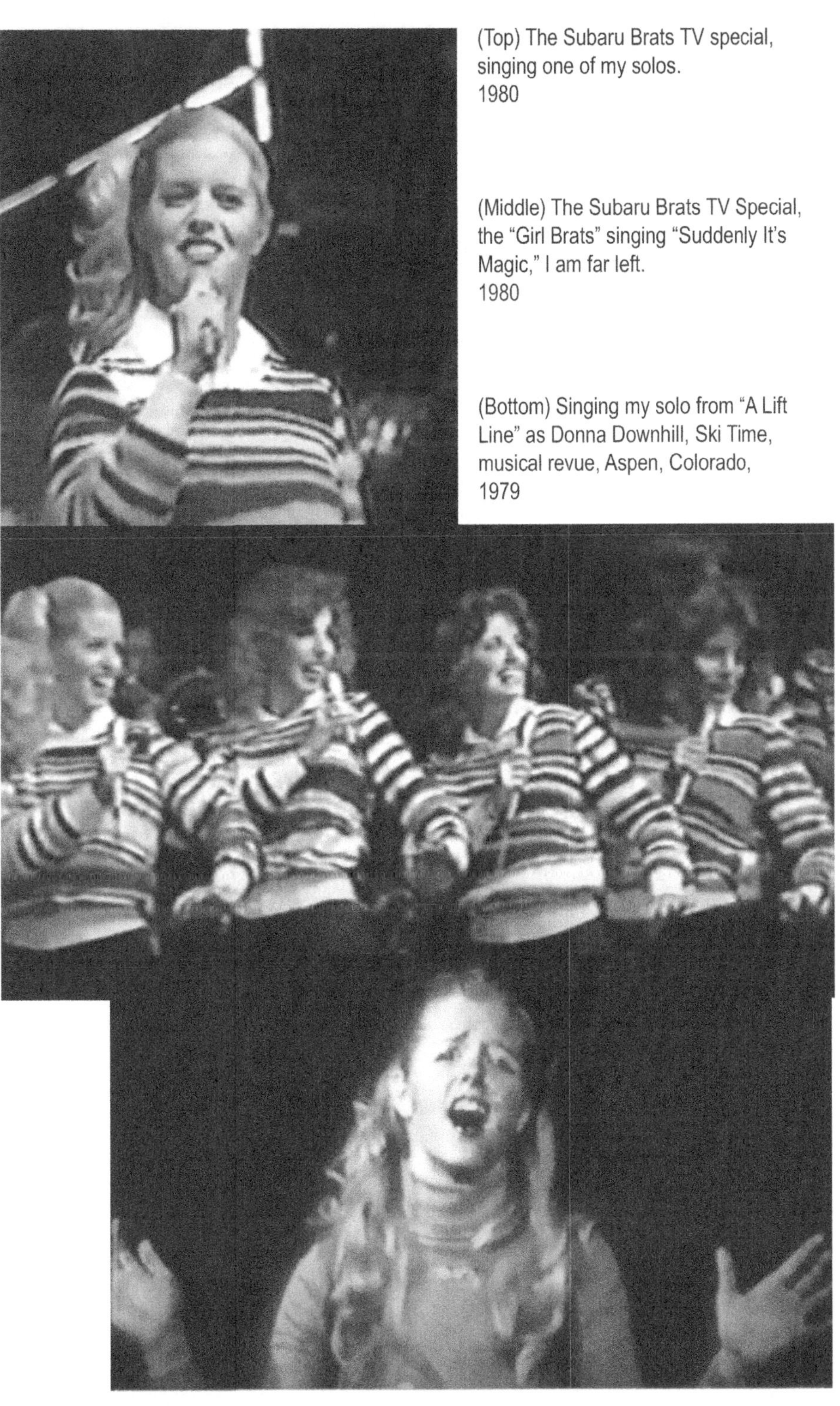

(Top) The Subaru Brats TV special, singing one of my solos.
1980

(Middle) The Subaru Brats TV Special, the "Girl Brats" singing "Suddenly It's Magic," I am far left.
1980

(Bottom) Singing my solo from "A Lift Line" as Donna Downhill, Ski Time, musical revue, Aspen, Colorado,
1979

VIVA LAS VEGAS, *Oct. 31, 1980*

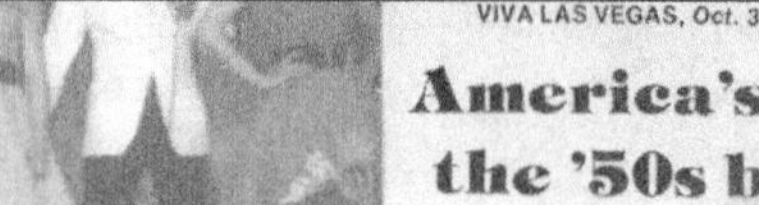

America's romance with the '50s brought to you by american bandstand's dick clark

'50s rock 'n roll

by Ira David Sternberg
Viva Las Vegas Editor

You don't have to remember the 1950s to enjoy it. But it probably helps. Either way, you're in for a fun evening at the "Nifty Fifties" revue, currently at the Marina Hotel and Casino.

The "Nifty Fifties" is a Dick Clark presentation, and the master of Clearasil make an appearance opening night with his wife and world-famous (if you follow "American Bandstand") Justine.

Danny and the Juniors put on a spirited performance, bringing back their classic "At The Hop," along with their 1958 hit, "Rock And Roll Is Here To Stay." The essence of 1950's music is fun and D and the J's bring out their element in the audience.

The dancers are dressed in appropriate dresses of the decade as they sing and dance their way through, including "Charlie Brown," "Rockin' Robin," "Johnny Angel" and "Get A Job."

The nifty fifties is a combination of sights and sounds of the decade, featuring Carl Waxman.

Interspersed between Waxman's monologue (some funny comments about the 1950s), Danny and the Juniors, and the Nifty Fifties dancers, are some hilarious filmclips, including scenes from "American Bandstand," and well-remembered commercials from the fifties, including Brylcream, Mr. Clean, Colgate and Edsel.

While the show start off slow, it builds fas and fun, music an memories for everybody. Even if you don't remem ber the fifties.

The "Nifty Fifties" a the Marina Hotel offer two shows nightly, p.m. and midnight.

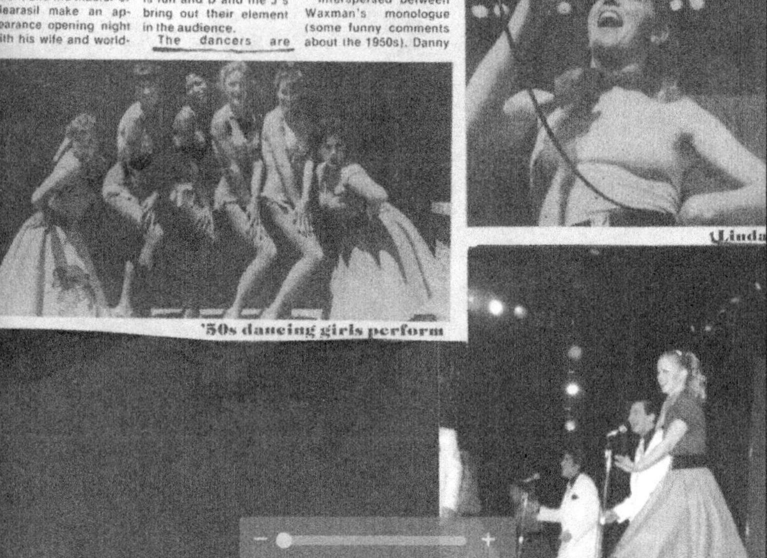

'50s dancing girls perform

Linda

(Above) me, middle right, with microphone in my one Las Vegas Show, *Dick Clark's Nifty Fifties*, 1980

CHAPTER TWENTY-ONE

GREASE IS THE WORD AND THE MOVIE

Grease was a relatively new musical that had opened on Broadway that I had done a bootleg production of at my Performing Arts college right before I left to go pro. I mentioned in an earlier chapter that I had learned how to twirl a baton for the part of cheerleader, Patty Simcox.

I called my agent and told him I had done the role, and I'd sure like a chance at the movie version, PUHLEASE! He supposedly tried to get me an audition, but could not, and I was quite frustrated at that. But guess who did the audition and won the part of Patty Simcox? My sexy girlfriend, Susan Buckner. And believe it or not, she was the only entertainment friend I was ever jealous of.

If you were born on March 13th, according to my astrological profile, you did not suffer from jealousy, and I was blessed not to have that character trait. Once I knew that I could not get the Patty Simcox role, I decided to go to a cattle call for chorus dancers that was posted in *Variety,* where most of the legit supporting dancer/singer roles were posted back then.

Cattle calls were sort of fun to go to, as hundreds of men and women showed up whether they were the correct type or not. The preferred type was always posted in the ad, for example: Female dancers wanted for the movie *Grease,* who can play high school age. Please dress as 50s era teenagers (which was what they wanted you to do for this one). Usually, you just wore dance rehearsal leotards and tights, and brought your dance bag full of dance shoes, water bottle, towel, etc. We had to dress in character for this one.

It was really like a big reunion of all your dance friends. The thing that always made me laugh and saddened me at the same time, were the old women, never men, that would come and audition. Some were in their 50s and 60s, who put on a lot of makeup, and dressed as required, to audition. It was kind of like Barry Manilow's song about Lola the old showgirl in the song "Copacabana." Oftentimes, at the beginning of the call they would put us in long lines and go down the rows and say stay or thank you, to save time and energy. If they said thank you, you picked up your stuff and left.

A bunch of us went together dressed as best we could as "Greasers" or "Pink Ladies" in poodle skirts. I wore my long hair in a ponytail, my satin jacket over a leotard top, a scarf tied around my neck and rolled-up capri jeans, with Capezio jazz flats. My girlfriends were similar, except one had a poodle skirt.

The choreographer was Pat Birch, who'd choreographed the Broadway show. We learned the "hand jive" dance that I already knew, plus a couple of other steps thrown in as a large group, and then we were split into groups of about eight, in two lines.

You'd do the routine once with four in front and then switch, front to back and do it again. We were all in one group of eight, and after we did it twice, we were ALL told thank you. It was shocking that not one of us got kept! We did bring cameras and took pictures of ourselves dressed up, as we'd gone to the trouble to do so.

The next day we found out that Pat Birch cast some of her dancers from NYC for the skeleton crew, the sixteen or so gals and guys that would make up the chorus parts along with the principal parts, so she was not looking for that many for the big dance sequences.

But then we got calls from our friends Susan Buckner, and Judy Sussman who was skeleton crew, who told us that Pat Birch had lost her list of needed chorus dancers from her L.A. cattle call, and we had the job of dancing in the prom sequence if we wanted it, for eight days of shooting. There was one catch: The female dancers had to go and find 50s prom dresses from thrift stores and wear those for the job. Paramount Pictures had run out of 50s dresses, but they had suits for the boy dancers.

Also, producer Allan Carr had worked out a deal with SAG, a special "Dancing Extras" contract and pay would be $110 a day. Dance work was usually about twice that, but Allan Carr was a wheeler-dealer, and it was what it was.

My brain went into high gear about the prom dress search, and I called my mom in Washington State and said, "Ma, I need you to send me all your old prom dresses hanging in your closet from high school for a movie I'm in with some girlfriends, and you will get to see them in the movie! Have Stan (my 13-year-old brother) help you. I'll pay for the postage, and I need you to do this quickly, like tomorrow or the next day, as the movie job starts in another week." SO, SHE DID! They came in a large wardrobe packing box and there were about five with poufy skirts.

I chose my dress first of course, then called three or four other friends of mine that I thought they would fit. The one I chose was not my favorite, that went to my girlfriend Chris Wallace. It was a satin dress, white with big red flowers, but I was so skinny for it. I had to wear my mom's freshman dress from 1948. It was the smallest, pink with a chiffon skirt. Three other friends took the rest, and when I watch the prom sequence I always look for them.

When you shoot a movie, you usually work from about 7am to 7pm, unless it is a night shoot. Like shooting a soap opera, that is all you do until it is finished, and why I liked episodic TV shows or stage shows the best—you actually had a life.

We rehearsed the dances for the prom sequence for two days and shot for the next six days. It takes longer to set up shots for film, often using a dolly, cranes, or handheld shots.

Chris Wallace and I carpooled as we lived fairly close to one another, and we had great talks going down to the old high school south of Los Angeles.

We hung out with Susan in her trailer instead of being in the big cafeteria all day long. Susan was having an affair with the hot hot hot Jeff Conaway, a well-publicized story, so if the trailer was rockin', don't come a knockin'.

I found a sweet young brunette guy for a dance partner. He could lift me with my hands on his shoulders into a handstand, and my dress would fly over me, but it wasn't shown in the movie.

People always ask about John Travolta, and here is my story: We were taking a break from filming one day, and I was sitting on the floor like a little pink flower with my pink chiffon skirt spread in a circle around me. John was standing about ten feet away from me, and our eyes met and didn't move for the longest time. John's best feature was his gorgeous blue eyes. However, I felt he had a long neck and photographed better than his appearance in person. We never spoke and that was our unspoken connection. I never met or even got close to Olivia, but she noticed me, and I will talk about that later.

The eight days came and went, and I was glad when it ended. I was a bit of a whiner on this gig. It was summertime, and shooting in the gymnasium was very uncomfortable, and I was bored a lot of the time.

I was asked to do the finale scene at the fairgrounds a week later, but gave the job voucher to my girlfriend, Charkie. I must say, when we couldn't do a job, we'd try to offer the work to each other. The on set atmosphere was definitely relaxed, as she mentioned bringing a full cooler of beer to the set every day, as there was very little dancing, mostly just running around the fairgrounds, playing with the games and rides.

The movie was a HUGE, MAJOR MOTION PICTURE MEGA HIT. Some people cannot believe I was in it when I tell them, but I have my mom's prom dress on display in my house, with a framed screenshot of me doing the stroll line hanging on a wall, if you don't believe me!

Next, I did get one of those GOLD jobs where I did not have to audition. Slimy Jaime Rodgers called me for a TV special he was doing the following week called *The Magic of ABC*, a preview of some of the network's up and coming Fall 1977 TV lineup. I fit what he needed perfectly for one of the production numbers at the end of the special, and it was two weeks of work at about $700 a week, alrighty then!

A new young magician, David Copperfield, who was a brilliant large-scale illusionist, was the star of this TV special, introducing some of the ABC shows and stars. I had never worked for a magician before and only worked for one more after David. When assisting them, they are very, very serious, borderline uptight, because if you blow the trick for them, THEY look the fool. I had to sign a contract, as well, not to give his tricks away, but have told people throughout the years what to look for.

We rehearsed with David a lot, as we were very involved with him, and he danced as well. I was part of a trick with Hal Linden, who was behind life size playing cards, then came out on set behind them, then went up to the ceiling on a lift, and the cards dropped away, and there was Barney Miller!

Donny and Marie Osmond were guests on the show, and I assisted in sawing David in half in a black box, and when we'd finished the sawing, Donny had replaced David in the box. Then we did a cute dance number behind Donny, to his most recent hit, "You've Got Me Danglin' on a String," and we female dancers were dressed in gold foil hot pants outfits that were as cute as Donny. Donny was a doll and nice, while Marie seemed rather cold.

The entire supporting cast of dancers did a big grand finale production number from the musical *On the Town,* with David and two male dancers as sailors on leave in New York, with the female dancers as various characters, from hookers to society ladies to little girls (me). It was on a huge soundstage, and it was the hardest, most athletic dancing I'd ever done on TV. The end featured David levitating dancer Cindy Ashley on a painted landscape of NYC, in front of a painted Empire State Building, and then bringing her down into his arms. It was impressive.

A few weeks later, my good friend Bridget asked if I could sub for her, working for another magician who did some sleight of hand, and large-scale illusion for a live event on stage. For this type of work, you had to have a certain height and flexibility to squeeze yourself into small areas, but if you were too small, it'd be obvious what was going on. The height requirement was between 5'2" and 5'4" inches tall. I was 5'3" but people always said I looked taller because I was thin.

So, for $100, I rehearsed for about six days at the magician's home in his back yard. He had two young male assistants as well, so a cast of four. I learned the trick, "Stack of Boxes," where it started with one box and they built me, and I stepped out at four. Also, "Box of Swords," where I went down into a box, with swords stuck into the box, then opening it, revealing I'm gone, next pulling the swords out, as I'm revealed, standing up.

The big finale, "Glass Casket," was fairly nerve-wracking. I was in the bottom compartment of a large, long wooden box with glass over it. It was rolled out onto the stage and the magician threw a black sheet over the box and knocked on the box, when I pushed open half of the bottom section, threw my left leg over the other closed half, pushed the rest of my skinny body to the closed half, closed the other section and stretched myself out, as the assistants were slowly spinning the box around the stage.

One of them lifted the blanket to the back of the casket and stopped spinning it. The magician then pulled the black sheet off the casket in a TA DA-style sweep, and I am there, laying on my side, in my silver leotard with white go-go boots. I stepped out onto the stage floor, with the boys holding my hands, nodded twice to the applauding audience, and did a little sauté 'arabesque, and ran off the stage. Whew, I didn't fuck it up! Interesting to learn but once was enough.

At the beginning of March 1977, I was sent on an audition to play Arnold Horshack's sister on a spinoff of *Welcome Back, Kotter.* The fifth episode of *Welcome Back, Kotter* that season was shot as a pilot for Ron Palillo, who was to have his own show about his crazy, dysfunctional family. That's what I was reading for. The casting director really liked me and I was called back to read with Ron for the network. It was nerve-wracking, as I had to block and memorize my scene with him, but he was so very supportive and nice, and I was proud to have had this opportunity with him.

I did a good job, but I told my agent, "My God, I look nothing like him." But apparently Horshack's mom had had FIVE different husbands, and four more children, so I just had to be cute and likeable. Anyway, the spinoff was scrapped, so no Linda Horshack for me, though it was an awesome memory.

Al hadn't worked much since he came back off the road at the beginning of '77, and he wasn't getting many producing jobs, but he didn't seem that concerned yet. He resolved to not do any solo albums for a while, as the tour thing had not been lucrative, and he lost money. He'd also developed some new friendships.

One was Al's doppelganger named Dave, who was a road manager for various rock bands, and the other was Jeff "Skunk" Baxter of the Doobie Brothers, who was nick named "Skunk" because he didn't like to bathe. When they looked at me, they gave me the heebie-jeebie-creepy crawlies, if you get my drift, a woman's intuition bigtime.

It was around this time that Al started having boys' night out on Saturday nights. He had a custom-made pink suit, with a nice dress shirt and tie, and he'd clean up nicely and head on out the door, to hang with his two new friends, and who knows what else. I wasn't going to ask a lot of questions, but it made me think of the saying, "Idle hands are the devil's workshop, an idle mind is the devil's playground,"

Sometimes I'd go to a party without him with friends, or have friends over and we'd play music, dance, drink wine and watch the new and extremely popular late night TV show, *Saturday Night Live*. Thank God for that, and I'm still a fan, fifty years later.

On October 20th, we were awakened by a phone call around 7am as we lay sleeping in our custom made "Cleopatra's Barge" wooden bed. It was Al's part-time assistant, Elaine Angel, practically screaming on the phone to turn on the TV news. We saw a still shot of Lynyrd Skynyrd's latest album *Street Survivors*, with the band in front of fiery flames on the street behind them. The band had been in an airplane crash in a tree covered, wooded swamp in Gillsburg, Mississippi in their private leased plane.

There had been some fatalities, but the news wasn't saying who or how many yet. Al hung up the phone and said, "Ronnie's dead, I can feel it."

Ronnie Van Zant was the lead singer and front man. Of course, Al was right, Ronnie, along with the Gaines siblings, road manager Dean Kirkpatrick, and the two pilots. Lord have mercy! We just sat in bed and cried and cried, it was so heart breaking. The rest of the band survived, as did two backup singers and another road manager, but the tour they were on was cancelled, and their new *Street Survivor* album went platinum overnight.

Al got some of the details and decided to go to their memorials in Jacksonville, Florida, but I felt it best for him to go by himself, they were his band, his friends, and the ones I was close to, like Gary, were in the hospital. By then, we had a menagerie of pets: three dogs and two cats, and I had classes at USC, too, so I stayed home.

About six months later, Allen Collins came to the house by himself and told us the details of the crash: The horror of the plane going down into the trees that sounded like baseball bats hitting the airplane, everyone passed out or barely conscious and moaning, Artimus, the new drummer running to a farmhouse through the swamps to get help (he was in the best shape, and a health nut), the two pilots hanging in the trees near the airplane dead, one wing on top of Gary Rossington breaking a hundred bones in

Gary's body, and lastly socks and underwear hanging in the trees like decorations from all the impacted suitcases. As it was, Allen had come within a quarter of an inch of his neck being broken and he had to have his body and head taped to a stretcher to make it to the hospital.

It took several years, but the remaining band members did pull themselves together and formed a new Lynyrd Skynryd band, with Johnny Van Zant, Ronnie's younger brother as lead singer, and Gary Rossington as their leader until he passed. They are continuing to tour to this day, forty-eight years later, although all the original members have passed away now. They are considered one of the best rock bands in my lifetime and although I never saw any of them again, except Allen, they are part of my DNA, along with the Tubes, and I will see them all again in the next life.

Good old Ray Anthony had called me just before the plane crash to do a brief gig for him that I accepted. It was three weeks in Mexico City, and a little touring outside of the city. I had said yes, as Al wasn't going anywhere, and could look after the pets. It began the second week of November, perfect timing before Christmas, too, as I was going home to Washington for Christmas to be with my family. It would be a nice break for me to get away from the Skynyrd tragedy.

We were in Zona Rosa in Mexico City, at a hotel with a show room called the Alexandria. Zona Rosa was the upscale Beverly Hills-like section of the city, so it was lovely, and we had nice rooms at the hotel.

I was with some new Bookends who I'd never worked with before, but we quickly got our parts figured out. I became friends with one of them, Rhonda Miller, a cute blonde who could dance but not sing, so Ray just let her mouth the words, while the rest of us carried the singing. Ray allowed her to do that as he had an eternal crush on

Rhonda, who he'd also sexually harassed, but Rhonda was married back then, with a big muscular husband, so he left her alone.

We had some fun times. We went to the National Museum of Mexico on a day off, and it was soooo wonderful. There was a huge Egyptian section, and some of Frida Kahlo's original paintings.

We also did a Mexican television variety show starring a man called the Walrus, a mature man with a white moustache and beard that made him look like a walrus. We did our 40s medley and about half the band played behind us.

We then went to Taxco on our other day off, as Ray had booked a one-nighter there on a terrible outdoor stage we could barely dance on. Taxco, at that time at least, was the silver capitol of Mexico, and I bought Al a necklace and one for me that I still have. Both were solid silver.

Rhonda and I were hungry after the shows, and the only convenient place where we could grab a bite after the show was at the local Denny's, so we would go there together. As blondes, we drew intense attention—every brunette head turned and stared at us, even as we ate.

On one of the last nights, as we were walking home from the Denny's we passed an alleyway and glanced into it and a man was in a trench coat flashing us!!! We screamed and ran and then laughed, as nothing happened and we made it to the hotel safely. It was the only time I was flashed my entire life. Viva Mexico!

I went back to La La Land for about ten days and then flew home to Bremerton for two weeks. My sister did, too, and we had a blast with my grandma, mom, and brother. Al was Jewish, so it didn't bother him, and he didn't even celebrate Hanukkah, so he didn't mind. He could enjoy his boys' night out, and I could see not only family but friends, too.

I had brought my skis home and a bunch of us went skiing at Crystal Mountain. Our friend, Bart Bruckman, was running it and let us sleep on his living room floor for an overnight. Then it was back to Bremerton for New Year's Eve at various people's houses, before going back to L.A. and what would be quite a different year.

CHAPTER TWENTY-TWO

i TURN 25 AND TiME FOR CH CH CHANGES

1978. Well ... bring it, right? The front lobe of my brain would be fully developed on my birthday in three months, and I was starting to feel differently about things. My career was chugging along just fine, my relationship, not so much.

I'm glad I went back to college at USC as I always liked learning, and I took a wonderful sociology course called "Marriage and Family interactions" that made me focus more on what I wanted from my partner. I never wanted children that much, partially because my poor mother had to struggle with the help of her parents to raise us, as her two husbands did not work out for her and she always swore that it affected her bi-polar mental illness, made it worse.

I loved animals, as well, better than kids and many people in general, but Al didn't even help me with those much, and I could've used more help with the dogs, but I fed, watered, and bathed them at least. While the two cats were always inside, Al would not allow the dogs in the house, and they got lonely. Not only that, we had coyotes in Coldwater Canyon.

I just started to feel like I didn't really have a boyfriend anymore. Our sex life had diminished greatly, and we never DID anything anymore at all. We didn't go to the movies, no concerts, no dinners out, pretty much no nothin'.

I did think it was partially because Al had gotten into debt from the album tour, but he was too proud to say as much. I also switched agents for movies and TV work as I felt Bill Meiklejohn had done as much as he could for me.

I got another good agent, Ray Sackheim, in Beverly Hills. But shortly after I got him, he was in a car crash and laid up at home for a long time. The agents that took over for him also did what Bill did: put me up for major motion picture roles as the star against the established stars, although I asked them to consider supporting roles first. You have to walk before you run. But once again, it fell on deaf ears.

The really funny thing, though, was that one of the agents there handled Mark Hamill, her *Star Wars* client, and she'd soon be quitting the Sackheim group to manage him, per his wishes.

When I brought some new headshots into the office, Mark was there and he walked up to me about two feet away and just stared at me smiling, a funny way to flirt, saying nothing. I smiled back but also said nothing and then excused myself. Mark wasn't really my type, and he'd also gotten in a car accident and despite surgery, his cute face was rather compromised.

I wasn't booking many acting jobs—a couple of print modeling jobs for Carl's Jr. as a counter girl, and another for a real estate company, and a Schlitz Beer Garden commercial that was a regional buyout. I'd also decided not to audition for any dance jobs for a while, just take my two or three dance classes a week.

Then I saw posted on the bulletin board at USC that Stephen Sondheim's "Follies" would be the yearly spring musical. I'd always wanted to do the show. I LOVED the book and the music, so I auditioned and got the role I wanted as Young Salley Durant—I wasn't old enough-looking to play old Sally. But I was just thrilled to be in the show. The rest of the cast was super talented, and many went on to be working actors. I had a wonderful time performing and had some strong singing parts that I was ready for. USC had a lot of money to put into production, and we had marvelous sets and costumes, and I got some flattering reviews in the newspapers as well.

I also had a couple of minor but physical affairs with a couple of college cuties from the musical and classes, and I was not happy with myself, or my personal life. This is NOT what I wanted, even though Al was fine with an open relationship. I wanted a committed physical relationship, and not hiding things, sneaking around, and possibly a family in the future.

It was June of '78 and I sat Al down and told him about my feelings, and he told me he wouldn't change. I wasn't mad, I just sort of felt nothing for him anymore, as for me there was no future for us.

I requested that I stay in the house through the end of the summer as it got hot, of course, and I wanted to use the pool. But I also needed that time so I could find a place to live and figure out my next agenda. He felt that was not unreasonable, so that was the plan. Al's manager, Stan Polly had had Al and me sign a pre-nup to protect both of us should we part ways wherein I'd get $10,000 and my 280 Z car.

I swear the universe has always looked out for me, and as luck would have it my dancer/Bookend friend Valerie

Miller was touring on the road with Bob Fosse's *Dancin'* and was subletting out her two-bedroom, two-bath apartment in the Wilshire district. One of our other girlfriends was paying a small amount to keep some clothes and possessions there but was basically living with her boyfriend who'd later become her husband, so I'd have it to myself, at least to begin with.

Then I get a phone call out of the blue from Joe Cassini, the Krofft choreographer, my favorite choreographer, to be in a TV special for the Kroffts for a band called The Bay City Rollers who I had heard of but was not really into.

They were a teeny bopper band from Scotland who wore a lot of tartan clothes and had very catchy, poppy songs. The Kroffts had an entire 13-week series that they contracted them to do on Saturday mornings for the young girls and little kids. The TV special was the pilot to the series.

I had to start working again as I'd have pay rent and utilities, so I said you betcha and thank you. And a BIG PLUS ... two of my close girlfriends, Bridget Hollomon Johnston and Susie Guest, would be on it with me, with only two other dancers who I didn't know. Joe also said that he'd give me some featured dance/acting parts which he did, but requested that I partner with the frontman/ lead singer Leslie McKeown, as he was a handful with an attitude problem. I said, "Yah, I'll kick some Scottish ass if I have to." Uh huh, done deal.

Now this was about the middle of August. I had a place to live, I'd already started packing up some of my stuff, all I had furniture-wise was a chest of drawers, so it wasn't going to be difficult.

Most of you who've gone through a substantial living together or marital breakup know that if you have pets or kids, that is really the most painful part of it. No kids of course, but there were the two cats and three dogs. We had acquired Bozo and Bebe, our part German Shepherd and full breed German Shepherd from various giveaways, and they were such sweet dogs. I had taken Bebe to obedience school and really enjoyed it—she did not need obedience, but she was shy and needed self-confidence.

My sister Kathy had been with Sheik Walid El Jufali through college, but they had graduated in 1977 in San Diego, part of the USIU system that also had my performing arts college. They decided to part ways, although Kathy could've married him and moved to Saudi Arabia and been filthy rich, but the lifestyle wasn't for her, and I was relieved.

Kathy and Walid had an Afghan Hound, Manfred Manny, that Kathy couldn't keep, as she was getting a small apartment and downsizing from what she and Walid had had. So, Al and I took Manny, and he was a sweet, beautiful dog. I liked to take him to USC with me to rehearsals for *Follies* and show him off.

Anyhow when I knew I was leaving Al, I was talking to my manicurist and told her I didn't know what to do about him. Al said he would keep Bebe and Bozo and our black cat Snarflee, and I would take our Bluepoint Siamese, Archie. Al loved Snarflee (a made-up name by him) cuz he ate pop rocks, and he'd bought Archie from a pet store for me, and I could take him with me. My manicurist came to the rescue for me as she had a doctor who was Middle Eastern who had been wanting an Afghan Hound. He had a nice home and a large yard, and I trusted her. I brought Manny down to the salon and tearfully watched him drive away with her. I'm tearing up writing this.

CHAPTER TWENTY-THREE

THE BAY CITY ROLLERS

The Bay City Rollers were about as Scottish as one could imagine and a fabricated group like The Monkees, but younger, at least when they started in 1971. They were from Glasgow and Edinburgh and were discovered by a sort of shyster/grifter and a convicted child sex offender named Tam Paton, but he was brilliant in putting this band together and promoting them.

It took them until 1975 to really get touring and become worldwide teeny bopper sensations, with their platform shoes and tartan clothing, and they were cute. They got their name from Bay City, Michigan—they threw a dart at a map of the United States and that's where it landed. And they liked rollers better than rockers—it just sounded, well, better.

We walked into the first day of rehearsal, and it was so good to see my girlfriends and Joe Cassini and his nice and wonderfully talented assistant choreographer, Casey Cole, who had been his assistant on the many other TV shows I had done for the Kroffts.

Over on the opposite end of the room were the Bay City Rollers with sort of strange looks on their faces. We were introduced to them, and I think we shook their hands. For whatever reason, we didn't start dancing right away, so Bridget, Susie, and I started goofing around imitating Jaime Rogers teaching his dance classes with a lot of jumps with contractions and rolling on the floor, just having one of them there good times. I think the band was fascinated by our antics, maybe even scared.

We didn't think they were very good looking ... yet. Some had bad teeth, but they all had nice hair and they were thin except for Eric, who was on the chubby side—but he had the cutest face. So, we were assigned our partners and yes, I got the lead singer, Leslie or Les. He started talking to me and I couldn't understand a word he said, but he was amusing himself and laughing. His Gaelic accent was so thick, I just smiled and tried to laugh when he was laughing to be polite.

We were dancing with them to a 50s rock & roll medley which would be the finale. We rehearsed with them for about an hour. Then it was time for a meal break. The girl dancers all went to lunch and discussed the fact that we could not understand what our partners were saying, and how could they be teen idols when they weren't very good looking? Then we came back from lunch and learned our opening dance routine to their big hit "Saturday Night," with pom poms, a cheerleader-like routine as there was a cheer in the song: "S-A-T-U-R-D-A-Y NIGHT".

I went home to Al as I was still living at Freebird Mansion, and he asked me if any of those Bay City Rollers were touching me? I was sort of surprised at the question as we were splitting up and so what if they did? But my reply was, "We have to do some simple partner work with them so yes, when we partner them, I have to do so," and that was that with no further questions.

The next day began with sitting around waiting for the Rollers to get done doing a music rehearsal. Bridget had brought a MAD magazine. So, Bridget, Susie, and I sat on the soundstage in the audience chairs placed for the fans on taping day and read it and laughed our collective asses off, I hadn't read MAD in years! Such hilarious writing and cartoons.

We also put guest stars Eric Estrada and Scott Baio, who was twelve years old, into the finale with the Rollers, as was the Krofft tradition for a musical variety finale. Eric Estrada seemed to want attention from the female dancers, but we were not interested, and Scott Baio was quite shy having to do a version of "hand jive" with me on top of a vintage car.

Day three of rehearsals were going along well for us girls, and we could understand the Rollers better now. Leslie told me that they hadn't wanted to do this TV series but Tam, their manager, got good money for it and it would broaden their fan base in the USA. But Leslie was leaving the band after this final pilot special was done filming and embarking on a solo career. It had created tension between him and the rest of the band—that is why he was being looked at as difficult to work with.

Day four was just polishing the routines, but I found myself looking forward to seeing Leslie (don't tell Al). Day five was taping day and what a wild scene with the fans' Rollermania.

I think I may be one of only a few hundred living souls that witnessed BOTH Beatlemania and Rollermania LIVE, up close and for real. In 1964 when I was eleven years old with my mom and sister in Seattle at Key Arena with Beatlemania, and this taping day in August of '78 as a twenty-five-year-old professional dancer for the Bay City Roller TV special.

We were all getting into our costumes in the dressing rooms back behind the set and hanging with the Rollers. It was obvious that four out of the five of us had developed crushes on our partners, despite being in a relationship or even married. They were basically nice young men, and we were all sorry the week was at an end. ALL of us made plans for lunch the next day at Casa Cugat on La Cienega, not that far from KTLA, so it wouldn't be a hassle for the Rollers. I, personally, was starting to fall in love with mine, Leslie.

The Krofft's started the filming off with the band in a limo coming into the alley behind the studio and had alerted some of the female teenage fans to be there. So that is how the TV special started, the band pulling up and teenage girls jumping all over their limo and them coming out and barely avoiding getting mauled. It then switched to them running into the soundstage where several hundred teenage girls were already seated in the audience behind some rather flimsy drywall barriers, which some proceeded to push down.

We were standing in front of them getting ready to dance the opening number "Saturday Night." It was scary, as we could've gotten injured by the falling walls. The shot was stopped, the dry wall barriers were put back up, and the Rollers re-entered the soundstage and as soon as the lyrics began, we came running out with our pom poms and our cheerleader-style dance.

Then the dancers took a break, and the Rollers did some jokes and banter in front of the sometimes-screaming teenage female audience. Lunch was called after that, and then we finished up the finale with Eric Estrada, Scott Baio, the two "little people," Patty White and Billy Barty, the Rollers and the dancers. I got some very good roles as promised and got to dance with Leslie again as my partner. The end of one of the segments had me sitting on his knee, and he gently bit my neck playfully to my delight. Yes, we were smitten.

After finishing the shoot, Leslie, Eric, and Woody invited us to go for some hors d'oeuvres and some wine at an exquisite wine bar on Sunset, and Bridget and I joined them. It was then that Leslie invited me to come and visit him at L'Ermitage, his hotel in Beverly Hills. I said I couldn't that night, but maybe in the next couple of days.

The next day we had lunch, the Rollers treat, at Casa Cugat—the five dancers, and only four of the Rollers, (as Derek Longmuir, the drummer, was a bit anti-social or not into women or some such thing), and we had a great time. Once again, Leslie said he'd be home that evening and to please stop by. I told him I had an acting class, which I did, but maybe afterwards around 8pm. I went home and changed my clothes, went to my acting class for ninety minutes, as I loved Michael Verona and my class, then headed straight to L'Ermitage.

I knocked on the door of Leslie's room and he opened it, grabbed me and pulled me inside. We began with passionate kissing, and then straight to the bedroom, almost ripping each other's clothes off. Leslie had a bottle of baby oil by the bed which he preceded to gently rub all over my breasts on down, and then on himself, and it was very slippery and an exotic new lovemaking experience for me, especially since I had not had sex with Al in quite some time. But I was still living with Al, so after a quick shower I had to get home. I decided driving home that I would start moving out sooner than the end of the month, as Valerie's apartment was available anytime.

I wanted to continue to see Leslie and I could do so only if I was truly single. So that is what I did. I didn't really tell

Al why, I just said I felt it was time, but I'm sure he probably knew something had happened between me and one of the band members. He didn't ask, and I didn't tell.

I took my Blue Point Siamese cat, Archie, my Z car, the clothes on my back, the clothes in my squished little closet, one painting that was a Jerry Williams piece I'd bought for myself and left. Valerie's apartment was only about fifteen minutes away, so it was relatively easy. I had no furniture except a small chest of drawers from another friend who brought it to Valerie's.

Ironically my sister Kathy had applied to USC's law school, had been accepted, and needed a place to live. She had stayed in San Diego for a year after graduating with a B.A. in political science and won a full scholarship/ fellowship to the law school, one of only two awarded in 1978. I had taken a leave of absence from USC as I needed to work again. I also told Al that he only had to give me $5,000 instead of $10,000, as I felt sorry for his financial situation.

The next time I saw Leslie, he came over and stayed two days with me as he moved out of L'Ermitage and just had a couple of suitcases of clothes in the living room. He had to go back to London, before he went to Japan, for a solo tour and recording a solo album, but the plan was that in about two weeks we'd go on holiday somewhere together before he went to Japan.

So, he left, and the next day I had an audition for an acting role in a religious film, *The Investigation*, produced by Family Films. It was for the role of Mary, a modern-day Mary Magdalene who was a reformed porn star, working in a downtown L.A. soup kitchen. The plot involved this nice-looking middle-aged man driving all over the city looking for Jesus, in modern day present times. He was working with the government, as they were trying to hunt down Jesus. He visits rich people and poor people, who Jesus had been known to hang out with, but the government found Jesus first and executed him.

He came to the soup kitchen to ask why she'd quit the sex worker business to help the poor. The character had a full ten sentence monologue explaining this to the investigator, and she goes upstairs in the soup kitchen to discuss her story and his search.

So, here's the deal on this: I got the part. We shot at a real soup kitchen with real needy folks in downtown L.A. and that part was fine. L.A. was having a heat wave, and the room upstairs was showing 105-degrees on a thermometer. One fan was going but it was stifling, and I felt like I might pass out but said nothing.

My director was an Episcopalian priest, not a professional director, and he let me say my monologue directly to the camera as an aside, like Mathew Broderick did in *Ferris Bueller's Day Off* for shits and giggles. WRONG! It was the longest day of filming in my life, and such a disappointment as I'd finally won a co-starring role on a movie.

I got though it without passing out, but when I went to the premiere about a month later, the visual part of my monologue had been cut completely, only the audio played to the lead actor's face as I spoke it. (I am so sorry I do not recall his name.) I was retained in a couple of brief scenes before and after that scene visually, but my monologue was all gone.

The next day, however, I was flying to Honolulu to see Leslie, such a nice reward. He had called me the week before and told me that was the logical place to go as it was tropical, gorgeous, and on route to Japan. Super fine with me, I just wanted to see him ANYWHERE! A ticket would be waiting for me at Hawaiian Air at LAX, and my sister would be home and take care of my cat, Archie.

A five-hour plane ride later, and I am met by my new boyfriend with a beautiful floral lei, and passionate kisses. We grabbed my suitcase and Leslie said, "I've got a surprise for YOU." We didn't go out to where the cabs are, we went to the back of the airport, to the tarmac, and there awaiting us was a helicopter with a private pilot. "He'll be taking us to the North Shore to Turtle Bay, and The Ritz Carlton Oahu, but first, a ride to look at the Island," he joyously informed me.

I'd never been on a helicopter, so how exciting for me, and it was! Although I'd seen the beauty of the Island from my previous trips, this was a magnificent view of paradise as my new boyfriend held me tight beside him. There was a landing strip at the hotel, so we landed right there.

As we headed to our room, Leslie said that his friend, confident, and personal photographer from Germany—Booby was his name—who'd be joining us on this trip but mainly just for meals and drinks at night and sometimes by the beach and pools, but he had his own hotel room of course. Booby, I was to find out, was sort of a big brother figure to Leslie, as he was in his mid-thirties, and Leslie was two years younger than me—at twenty-three, the youngest beau I'd ever had at that point.

It was time for dinner, and there were some very nice restaurants at the hotel. We called Booby in his room to come and join us, and hey, I liked the guy. It was very pleasant and fun, and he added nicely to the conversation, not a third wheel at all.

Leslie and I spent a lot of time on the beach or at the pool. Leslie had also rented a VW Bug, and we went into Honolulu to eat at my favorite shabu-shabu restaurant and then back out to Turtle Bay. Leslie turned into a little kid on the beach. He had me bury him up to his neck in the sand, loved going into the ocean, and just sort of running on the sand and acting goofy. I could tell that having grown up in cold, wet Scotland (their summertimes sucked), this was paradise and such a treat for him. I was happy he was enjoying Hawaii so much.

Eight days passed quickly, and it was time for him and Booby to go on to Japan, and me to go home. Bummer, man, but Leslie assured me that he would call me a couple of times a week, at least from Europe, as he wasn't staying in Japan for more than three weeks. Booby had told me a few days earlier at dinner that he'd NEVER seen Les look at any other female like he looked at me, and I did see what he meant when we had to part ways. "I love you," Les told me, in his Gaelic Scottish Brogue, and I told him I loved him back. Booby took some great pictures of us that I still have to this day. Bye bye, baby, bye bye.

I got back to my sister and my cat, and Kathy seemed to be somewhat depressed. She'd purchased all of her law books for her freshman year at USC, and they were sitting by the staircase of the apartment. They reached up to my ribcage, about four feet high—big, thick law books full of cases, "so and so vs so and so," as I peeked in a couple of them. Lord have mercy!

My dancer gal pals were coming by a couple of times a week to see me and how I was getting along since leaving Al, and we were silly and frivolous at night, having a glass of vino or two. My sister had to go upstairs and study, and we did try to keep it somewhat quiet, hard when you're over the top silly. It was hard on my sister to concentrate and study those big, thick law books, what a drag.

Kathy comes home the following week and says, "I'm quitting law school, I want to dance like you." WOW, she's bailing on one of the only two scholarships/fellowships from the law school that year, worth how much? But she was in tears, and I gave her a hug and said, "That's okay, I wouldn't want to do it either," motioning towards all the law books. So, what are you going to do?

"Well, after I go to USC and bail and sell back my books, I'll just audition for dance jobs like you," was her committed reply.

Our mom had removed my sister from dance classes when she was ten years old as she was not going to them but instead running around with our teacher's daughter who was her age, stealing liquor and getting drunk, along with other crazy antics. Kathy had just started taking jazz and tap classes again in San Diego, the previous year.

My sister was always a brilliant tap dancer, as it's such a rhythmic, mathematical dance form, and my sister excelled at math. I couldn't control her—I was her sister not her mother. Now it just so happened that there was a big cattle call audition for a tap dance gig at the end of the week, so I invited her to come with me. I showed her how to dress, write a resumé, etc., and we got her a quick, cheap headshot.

It was for an HBO TV special that I knew my BFF Bridget would be in. The producers LOVED her, as she had done several HBO specials for them, and they loved her look, sort of retro/vintage, with a cute face and blonde hair. I didn't know that the producers were looking for a Bookend type to match her, and I'm not sure she really did either, but she already had the job, so she did not have to audition.

The show was called *Opening Night*, and it was all tap dance. It was being choreographed by Danny Daniels. He had done a lot of either tap or musical theatre-style choreography on Broadway and in film and television. He was about 50-ish, as far as I could tell. I had never auditioned for him before. He had a dance studio in Santa Monica where the audition was being held. He also had a tap dance troupe called *Danny Daniels' Dance America* that toured locally, and he was very, very serious about tap dance.

There were about 250 female tap dancers at the audition. We were all packed into his biggest studio that was used for *Dance America*. We all learned a tap combination. It was basic, and then we were put into groups of eight, standard practice. He moved us along fairly quickly, my sister and I in different groups. Kathy was first and was cut immediately and had to wait for me.

I was in a different group and got kept. Then I danced in the final group, and I was the ONLY tapper kept out of about 250 females. My sister was incredulous. We both didn't know it was because of my BFF, and what kismet was that? Danny Daniels was a talented genius, but also a serious, humorless man to work for. I did enjoy his choreography that was set in the past to ragtime music, with cute ragtime costumes. Better yet, I was with my BFF all day long!

I'm pretty sure he didn't like being told by the producers who to choose, and he did choose about four of his dance troupe females, who got no closeups, as the cameras were trained on Bridget and me. They just weren't that attractive. Bridget and I knew he didn't like having to hire either of us, and when we were on breaks, we made fun of the old curmudgeon and laughed our asses off. The Rolling Stones had just been on SNL with ripped T-shirts and parachute pants from "Beast of Burden," and we pretended Danny was dressed like them for rehearsal, a true visual. Danny would tell us to stop laughing, but it made us laugh more.

The sexy rock singer Eddie Money was one of the guests on the special and was performing live. We had finished all our dancing, and Bridget and I went to his dressing room and took a picture with him. I still have it! Then the producers asked Bridggie (her nickname) and me to sit in the front row of the audience and watch him, while he sang a cover of "You've Really Got a Hold on Me." Oh, hell yes!!! We did and they took some great shots of the two of us watching together, and it was a wonderful way for us to end the job, with our love of pop and rock music.

Leslie went back to his apartment in London after his appearances in Japan, which only lasted a couple of weeks. He had to call me, as he could afford the long distance, not me. He would call on Wednesday and Friday nights about 6pm my time. He was recording and writing a new solo album called *All Washed Up*, and he'd written a song about us called "Long Distance Love," which turned out to be repetitive, and sort of melodramatic, but sweet and flattering, nonetheless.

He'd say wonderfully romantic things like he was looking at the beautiful night sky and thinking of me, wishing I was there. I told him I wished I was with him, too. If he wanted me, I was certainly available. He didn't want the fans to see us together, as the paparazzi was everywhere, and he was in all of the teeny bopper magazines like *Tiger Beat* and *Teen Beat.* Since he split from the Rollers, he could not come back to the states for a while, as Clive Davis from Arista Records was out to slap a lawsuit on him for bailing on his contract from the band.

Now it's October, and I get a call from my girlfriend, Charkie Phillips, who has been hired to choreograph a segment of a TV special called *It's a Star Wars Christmas,* a one-day job and there was no dancing. We'd be in Wookie costumes as Wookie families and cast according to height. Charkie said my sister could do it, too, and day rate on it was $250 to just stand around in the Wookie costumes. So sure, that was a round-trip ticket to SEATAC airport for Christmas in Bremerton.

Two days later, we're on a soundstage in our Wookie costumes, with black around our eyes under our Wookie heads. Charkie separated us out into about five or six families of about three to five family members each. All we did was walk from stage right onto the set with our

Wookie family. There were four of us, with my sister as the mom, and another man as the dad, with me and one other person. My sister was 5'7" so she was the mom.

Shortly after we were taught our blocking, Mark Hamill, Harrison Ford, and Carrie Fisher came onto the set in their *Star Wars* costumes. My oh my, if Mark Hamill didn't come straight over to me and start staring at me with the Wookie head on! It was as if I was a magnet for him and he could find me anywhere, I swear! That only lasted about ten seconds, once again saying nothing, and then he left.

Our Wookie family was close to the small stage where the principals, along with R2-D2 and C-3PO, were to address us with some words of good will towards men. When we were rehearsing, Harrison Ford was carrying around a Coors beer, and drinking, and when he talked to people, he talked out of the side of his mouth. I was not that impressed. Carrie Fisher, however, sang a GORGEOUS Christmas song of hope and peace, and I loved her voice and watching her sing.

Those Wookie costumes were hot, and it was a warm early October day, and some were starting to complain about the heat. We were able to take our Wookie heads off and take a breather, at which time Mark Hamill, like a bad penny, came over again and just stared at me with my blackened eyes, and this time I just laughed out loud. I think he was hoping I'd say something to him, but nope I didn't say a word. Two could play that game. My sister and others were impressed at his antics. I just shrugged my shoulders and played dumb.

We got released early, as soon as they felt they had a good take of Carrie's song. We made our $250 day rate, the only time my sister was ever on TV, and it was rated as one of the worst TV specials of all time, LOL! The writing was inane and shameful, and I couldn't even watch the whole show when it aired on November 17th. I watched my part and turned it off. Hence, I call this story, *I was a Teenage Wookie.*

Next was an audition for Michael Kidd, the iconic movie choreographer, for a brief tap dance sequence in a new movie with George C. Scott, Ann Reinking, and my SPA college alum, Barry Bostwick. The title of the film was *Movie Movie.* It came only a few days on the heels of *The Star Wars Christmas Special and* would only last for a few days. It was just doing a time step over and over again, alongside character actor/comedian Red Buttons. He was a red-haired comedian who was a doppelganger to my dance teacher, Jack Tygett, except for the red hair. I went to the audition with my sister in tow again, but once again she did not book the job, but my friends Charkie and Bridget did, along with me.

The film took place in the mid 1930s, and we were dressed and had wigs on for that time period, and of the three of us, I looked the worst. The wig they put on me was dreadful, I looked like a cleaning lady. We didn't even rehearse the time step sequence, we just got into makeup, wigs, and costumes and Michael Kidd put us in a straight line to execute the steps with Red in front of us, yelling out some directions, fake directions, and then cut.

After that, we just hung out on the stage as ourselves doing crossovers and sitting on the stage. Red kept following me around and smiling in a sort of Mark Hamill flirting style, smiling and making goo-goo eyes at me all day long. If he were the last man on earth, he wasn't attractive to me, nor was Jack Tygett who did have some student relationships at school. Charkie and Bridget thought that the Red Buttons situation was hilarious, and I just thought to myself, why me? I was happy my girlfriends had a good laugh at my expense as I adored both of them.

The best part of this two-day gig for me was sitting on the stage, cross-legged as directed, and watching George

C. Scott do a minor scene with another actor who was an unknown. I tried my hardest to soak up his acting expertise by observation, but he was simply focused and natural. I made roughly $300 for the gig to use for Christmas expenses in Bremerton added to my teenage Wookie salary.

CHAPTER TWENTY-FOUR

ON THE ROAD AGAIN

I continued getting calls from Leslie twice a week, saying we loved each other, but after about three months, in November, I was losing any hope of seeing him again ever, and there were many complications.

I had heard long distance love affairs were painful, and I was in pain. My sister, meanwhile, had quickly learned that she was no match to most for the professional dancers she was up against at auditions. She didn't have enough ballet technique background that it required, so she started auditioning for some more second-rate jobs, and by golly, she got one!

It was a small animal circus that was going to tour Venezuela, as about as obscure as you can get. The director/ choreographer was a decent fellow with good English and a Latin accent. I went to a rehearsal that seemed on the up and up, and the choreography was okay. Ultimately, it was her decision. A girlfriend of hers from our hometown was also hired to dance with her. They were more like Vegas showgirl dancers who introduced the acts: pigs that jumped thru fiery hoops, dogs that hopped across the floor, cats that walked on tightropes, and chimpanzees with their hideous smiles doing various stupid animal tricks. No large horses, elephants or big cats.

They had both been staying at "Fort Shenandoah," which we nicknamed Valerie's apartment, in honor of those of us who had left their boyfriends and a place of strength to live there. It was also on Shenandoah Street, and that sounded like a name from some Western movie. Anyway, it all fits. Kathy and her friend left for Venezuela the first week of December, so I was all alone again at the "Fort" for wayward women.

I packed up my cat Archie and flew home to Bremerton for Christmas with my I Was a Teenage Wookie money, as planned. I had no one to take care of Archie and he needed to see my family. The friends I had left, who were still living in the area, all came truckin' over to see me, bringing wine and doobies, and it was a lovely Christmas.

I did hook up with a man who was really good looking, that I had dated for a while, and that was fun, and it told me what I already knew, and that was I didn't want to be committed to Leslie any longer.

I flew home after New Year's Day, and Leslie called the next day, and I told him I was in too much pain to continue to be committed to him. He said he was sorry, but circumstances didn't give him much of a choice. I told him to please keep in touch, that we could be friends. He was disappointed but said he understood.

I found out later that Les was two-timing me with his future wife, Peko Keiko, a Japanese woman he met in

London, who was a waitress at a Japanese restaurant. Les also had problems with his sexuality, drinking, and many financial problems with the management of the Rollers that would have been a nightmare for a wife, and I felt I really dodged a bullet by letting him go. I was done with rock stars after this.

I auditioned for the musical *Seven Brides for Seven Brothers*, in January of 1979. I had never seen it before, but I knew what it was about: Oregon territory in the post-Civil War era where there weren't enough women, and the men were competing to get the few there were. I was now free to go on the road after leaving Al.

My auditioners were Michael Kidd, yes, THE Michael Kidd, who choreographed the movie, Jerry Jackson, who would be the choreographer now, and a married couple were the two Canadian producers. Edwin Sherin would direct. He had also directed *The Great White Hope* on Broadway, and was married to actress, Jane Alexander.

We were also told that the stars of the show would be Jane Powell and Howard Keel, the stars of the film, twenty-six years earlier. HMMMM? I had worked with Howard at Music Circus in the summer of '74 in *Gigi*. He played Honoré, the mature gentleman who sings "Thank Heaven for Little Girls." I honestly wasn't quite sure who Jane Powell was, but I knew she was a movie star that did musicals.

The producers must have known what they were doing, right? And I just needed a job. So, after dancing, singing, and reading and Michael Kidd complimenting me almost to the point of embarrassment, I was given the job right then and there for the part of Sarah Kines, the second youngest bride.

We'd start rehearsals the beginning of the following week, and I had two girlfriends in the cast—Dorothy

Nichols from Music Circus, and Sha Newman from SPA, so that was great for me.

The whole cast was pretty darn nice and fun, and the dancing was very athletic for all of us. It had lots of exciting partner work and lifts, while wearing heavy fifteen-pound 19th century dresses made of heavy fabric, and petticoats.

I sweated as it was, but after our twelve-minute barn-raising "social" dance at the end of act one every night, I sweated off most of my makeup and had to reapply it at intermission. The seven brides, seven Pontipee brothers, seven suitors, assorted townspeople, and gymnast understudies were all doing just fine as a strong ensemble cast, but our stars were having some challenging times with each other, not to mention that the reviews and audience feedback was not complimentary—Howard looked too old, and Jane could not hit her high notes.

We were in Florida doing the well-known Kenley circuit of Orlando, Miami, and Fort Lauderdale, and I got to see many of my Hoxit aunts, uncles and cousins who had moved to Orlando and the Cocoa Beach area. My uncle Cecil had found work at the Kennedy Space Center. I had only met my one aunt, Lou. She had moved there along with her sister and Cecil, and some of their kids. They all came to see our show. During our stay, my friend Sha and I went on a tour of Cape Kennedy, and had dinner at their house in Cocoa Beach, a nice family experience for me.

Then we left Orlando for Miami, to play in a big barn of a theater. I came down with my first case of laryngitis EVER from coming into air-conditioned rooms, sweaty from dancing.

We did have understudies on the tour, but people told me to go and ask Howard and Jane if they had any tips for me to get over it quickly. I went to Howard first, and he overreacted when I whispered to him my question as to what could help my condition. He made a big deal about it like I was some sort of leper and said, "Stay away from me, I'm the star," and turned and almost ran away.

Laryngitis is stress-related and not communicable. So, I went to Jane, who, of course, was sweet as could be, and she advised just to rest my voice completely for the next couple of days, not even whispering, with hot tea and honey, and lots of water too. I recovered quickly.

When I worked with Howard Keel in *Gigi*, I don't think I had said as much as hello to him—certainly there was no conversation. When a well-known entertainer did ANY show back in the 70s and 80s, you were not introduced to them or unless you had a scene with them. In fact, professional etiquette dictated that unless the stars spoke to you, you didn't ask for autographs or pictures until the very last day you worked together, for the most part. But Howard and Jane were under stress from the reviews and feedback rolling into the producers.

They were both in their late 40s/early 50s and as I said, Howard looked old, and while Jane still looked young with her cute, petite little body, her voice was failing her on her high notes. Also, Howard said mean, derogatory things to Jane from time to time about her voice, bringing her to tears, trying to shift all the blame onto her for the harsh reviews they were both receiving. In the movie, they are supposed to be in their 20s, and they were just not pulling off the suspension of disbelief.

Our final city was Fort Lauderdale, and we had a wonderful four weeks at the Parker Playhouse. Also, Dorothy and I were invited to stay with my girlfriend Charkie's parents in the house that she grew up in. That would save us a lot of money.

When we took the bus from Miami to Fort "La De Da", as we nicknamed it, a carload of young men followed us into the city, pointing and smiling at the window where I was sitting. The cast got a big kick out of that, but nothing came of it.

What a beautiful city with the canals and pristine beaches. Mel and Sue Phillips were just the most fun hosts, and they came to see our show, and also had a party for the cast at their home. They took us to a couple of art galleries where I bought a numbered lithograph titled "Flying Cat Burger" by British artist Ronald Searle, that I have to this day.

The gay boys from our cast were staying at a gay hotel called the Marlin Beach Hotel, where they'd have afternoon tea dances and it was hilarious.

We were told this would be the end of our tour and this company of *Seven Brides*, as the producers didn't want to take it further and try and mount it on Broadway, as was their original thought. They thought people would just accept Howard and Jane, as the 1953 movie was so well received, but the reviews were just the opposite.

On the closing night of our show, the Marlin Beach Hotel threw a goodbye party for us. I was alone with the man who'd played my partner Frankincense aka Frank. We were in a corridor of the hotel for a few moments, and I got a very weird vibe from him, and how he was looking at me.

I haven't talked much about him, and I won't mention his name here. He was a very handsome man and good partner, but I felt he was rather unstable, so I did not get close with him, and he was also the boyfriend of one of the other brides.

We had one final matinee in our contract before we got on our flights home that night. When we said our goodbyes, my partner Frank told me that he had considered raping me that night before we parted ways, using that exact term and he was dead serious. My good God, I was then so glad our tour was at an end, and had it not been I would've had to talk to the powers that be about him, and that scared the hell out of me!

Back home to L.A. and Bridget, who had now replaced my sister as my roommate. She'd taken good care of my cat Archie, and I was grateful for that.

I saw an audition in *Variety* for a singing and dancing group of four young men and four young women for a possible touring group and TV special promoting the Subaru Brat. The ad said: "Must sing four-part harmonies and perform solos." I could do that. My voice had good pitch and vibrato, and my confidence in my vocal ability had grown.

I auditioned for it and got the job. I became one of the Subaru Brats, a prefab group with one original song, but mostly covers of old songs from the 1920s, and simple but hip dancing.

The arrangements had a modern twist, and we prerecorded them in a studio. The TV special had guest stars who the Brats would introduce vocally, in three or four-part harmony. I do owe Ray Anthony for the ability to do that.

Our guests were Helen Reddy, Vic Damone, and Robert Goulet. (We all held our breath as to whether he would show up or not.) Carol Larwence had divorced him (he had a well-known drinking problem), and he was living on his sailboat in Marina Del Rey. But he did show up, and he gave a fine performance.

We were also contracted to do an industrial for Subaru the day after the special, as it was the annual convention for the Subaru Dealers of America, and we were the entertainment on both days. We had to sing solos or duets, and I asked if castmate Brian Robert Taylor could sing "You're the One That I Want" from *Grease*, with me singing Olivia's part, and Brian singing John Travolta's part. He was handsome and brunette, and I was pretty and blonde, so it was perfect typecasting.

Ironically, we were rehearsing at Debbie Reynolds Studios in the San Fernando Valley at the same time that auditions were going on for the movie *Xanadu.* Brian and I had been in a smaller studio working on that song and goofing around, as Brian did a superb imitation of Burgess Merideth telling Sly Stallone, "You gotta chase the chicken," from *Rocky II*, as we laughed our guts out.

It was time for a break, so I went wandering around to Debbie's largest studio and looked in the open door to see a long table at the opposite end with choreographer/dancer Kenny Ortega and Olivia Newton-John sitting there. They were holding auditions for the movie, and they were on a break as well. I lingered in the doorway and saw Olivia say something to Kenny, as she looked at me. So, Kenny comes over to me, says hi, and asks what I'm doing there.

"Rehearsing for a TV special that I'm co-starring in," I say. "Well, would you like to be one of Olivia's muse sisters and tap dance with her in this new movie she's starring in?" he said.

"When would I have to start?"

"Next week," he grinned, and I said, "I'm taping this special next week and continuing rehearsals, could I start late?"

"No, that would throw the group dances off, but Olivia likes you. She LIKES you," with emphasis on LIKES.

"I can't quit this show, I like my producers and the Brats too much and I'm under contract, so thank her for me, but I just can't. When it rains it pours, huh? So sorry, Kenny!" I mournfully replied.

I never spoke to her when I was doing *Grease* in '77, but I guess she noticed and remembered me, and I sort of hummed to myself, "She likes me, she honestly likes me, she honestly LIKES me!"

The next week we shot the TV show and performed the morning performance live for the Subaru Convention.

We did a swell job on both, and especially for Subaru execs and their sales managers and wives.

For the TV show, it sure was a thrill to have our names announced one by one as we came on and see all our names in the credits. Up to that point they didn't do that. In the finale, there was also a huge group of about sixteen male and female dancers that did two large production numbers, many that I'd previously danced with on various shows. It was funny to see the way they looked at me as a singer, as many of them didn't sing, as in, "Why aren't you with US?" sort of looks.

After we did the taping and live show, the Brats were released from contract as they decided that we would not be the Brat Car Ambassadors, and we wouldn't get the Brat cars that we had hoped for. They were very cute little mini jeep cars, but all in all it was a good experience, decent money, and a good memory.

Back at home, my friend Bridget had not been working much, and that is always tough when someone you are living with is working and the other isn't. It's natural to compare yourself to the other person and ask yourself why you aren't winning the jobs.

Well, Bridget was a bit of a wild child, wilder than even me, and she also didn't sing. She had gone roller skating on the Venice boardwalk with a friend, high on acid, and fallen and broken her wrist. Skating under those circumstances was not a wise decision. I didn't like skating there because of the sand, and the LSD sure didn't make it easier!

My cute BFF Bridget had turned into a self-pitying whiner, and it was quite nerve-wracking to say the least. I had auditioned for another TV special for ABC and gotten chosen as well, by choreographer Ron Poindexter, who was a friend of Bridget's. But he couldn't hire her as her wrist was in a cast, which made matters worse. Valerie was also on her way home with *Dancin'* and it was her apartment, so I offered to move out to a place of my own. I was ready to be alone.

I found a small studio apartment on Laurel Canyon in the Valley near Ventura Blvd. I couldn't have a pet, so my friend Robert DeCapua, who liked cats, took Archie from me until I got a place where I could have one. I wasn't secure enough to get a larger place as this was decent and inexpensive. It had a cute A framed fireplace, too. I had next to no furniture, so I bought a bed, a chest of drawers, a papasan chair belonging to my sister, a TV, stereo, and a tiny table and chair for the kitchen.

Thankfully, there was a parking space out back for the Z car. I was much happier to be alone, but it was at this time that I learned that Al Kooper had been attending orgies, and I was devastated. Two of our mutual friends mentioned it to me, as they thought I knew, and I truly did not.

I guess that's what Saturday nights out with the boys was the past year and a half when we were still together. Al would get all dressed up, as the men had to put ties on the closed doors of the rooms they were in, to count how many men were in a room, as I later found out. I called Al and confronted him, and he had to admit it, but he was furious at our two friends for spilling the beans. I felt bad for them, since they didn't know that I didn't know. I stayed in the "hut" (the nickname my friends had given my apartment) and cried all weekend long.

Al did come over and see me and tried to make some sort of amends, even suggesting I go with him! He said if I took enough drugs, I'd enjoy it??? Enjoy a bunch of men I didn't know or even like sticking their VD infected penises in me or even touching my body? No sirree Bob, and it made me realize just how different we were in our views of sex, and that I would never get back together with him. I think he was probably a sex addict, which, back then, pre-AIDS, would be easy to become. L.A. was the porn capitol of the world at that time.

Now it was the summer of 1979, and I got a job down in Orange County for six weeks doing *The Music Man.* I had three other friends from the Valley in it, too. It was a 45-minute drive one way, and the four of us became quite close carpooling.

It was lovely, even though I hated the show itself (remember what Marge Tygett told you, again and again). I also wanted the role of Zaneeta Shinn, but I was cast as Gracie Shinn. I pulled a lot of focus anyway, and the producers really liked it. I didn't audition for Music Circus ingenue roles any more as another dancer who was my type had become friends with producer Howard Young and she got all the roles I could've played thru 1983.

CHAPTER TWENTY-FIVE

SKI TIME PLAYING IN THE ASPEN SNOW

Now it was Fall of 1979, and I'd gotten a letter from the Sackheim agency that I'd gone on the road too much last year and they felt they weren't able to send me on enough auditions, and they didn't make commission on my Equity stage contracts/shows since they did not book them for me. So be it. I still had my commercial agent and modeling agent, and they only wanted to put me up against established female stars that I couldn't beat out for roles anyway.

My girlfriend Coleen, the Playboy model, had also moved back to Florida, as she was close to her grandmother, and she wanted a more chill lifestyle and to go to college. I had a phone number of a man she had dated that took us both out to dinner one night, as he owned a company in town that made a lot of money, and he was a millionaire. A young-looking, long-haired fellow, nice-looking, with a nice personality, but she did tell me that he had a cocaine problem, like so many with money were having at that time in L.A. and all over the U.S.

Despite this, I decided to take a chance on this fellow, I had nothing to lose, right? I called him up and we both missed Coleen, although according to her they never had much of a serious relationship because of the coke use.

I told him I'd left Al, and he immediately asked me on a date. He wanted to go and see the movie *Alien* as it had gotten rave reviews from everyone who'd seen it and I was interested as well. He said I should meet him at his house near Malibu, and he'd drive in his car. So okay, I drive to his gorgeous home on a lush green private drive, meeting him after he got home from running his lucrative company.

He offers me a glass of Pouilly Fuisse the popular white burgundy that was the choice of people in the know at the time. So, I start to sip my wine, and then out comes the freebase pipe. "Let's just have a few hits of this before we go—have you ever done 'base' before?" he inquired.

"No," I said, but I've heard of it, knowing it was a form of cocaine. He shows me that you purify the coke through a strainer with liquid ether, and then you smoke the purified cocaine by lighting it on top of a coke pipe with a small blowtorch lighter. He does this and takes the first hit and then lights it for me. It was so strong, and it goes into your bloodstream immediately. It was a massive high, and we had a few more hits and then we actually made it out the door to see the movie.

We're sitting watching the movie *Alien*, plenty scary, and when the alien pops out of the astronaut's stomach I screamed out loud in the theater, I was so friggin' high. We did make it through the movie, but it was so intense, especially high on base.

We had to go back to his house as my car was there, and he starts up with the base pipe again, and more wine and that is how the rest of the evening went with freebase and wine, no dinner, no snack and we did get our clothes off but no sex.

Cocaine is a notorious threat to a man's libido, and his ability to get a hard-on. But we finally fell asleep with his sweet kitty and Italian greyhound asleep in the bed with us. He made us coffee so I could get home, as I felt pretty out of it from the debaucherous drug. I was also starving, but he had nothing to eat, and I couldn't wait to get out of there and home to some food.

He called me again the next day and asked me out to dinner, but I said, "PUHLEASE can we eat some dinner?" "Of course, no problem but come to the house again, six pm," he assured me. Okay, let's give it a try, once more into the breach, once more, and once more the same scenario: wine, freebase all night, no dinner, no sex and I smoked more cigarettes than I normally smoke to add to the unhealthy situation.

I wasn't really happy about the repeat situation, and I told him so, plus the freebase was so debilitating I was no good for anything except getting something in my stomach and laying around. If he called again, I was determined to turn him down, which he did do a couple of days later, and he said, "Let me make it up to you, come over and I'll make you dinner by candlelight. Do you eat meat?""

"Yes, on occasion but just so long as you make FOOD!" So, fool that I am I went a third time—third time's the charm, isn't it? The roast and potatoes were on the kitchen counter, the candles were on the dining room table bu, not lit yet.

"Let's just have some wine and just a couple of hits of base, and then I'll start cooking", he smiled. I should've flat out refused until AFTER dinner. I stupidly did not, and wash, rinse, repeat, no dinner, no intimacy, just the worst drug hangover I'd ever had. I almost crawled to my Z, barely got home, and was in bed almost all day, and that was truly the end of this man and freebase. It's a shame, and I'm sure a tragic statistic of some sort.

I had been auditioning from calls out of *Variety*, as there were always plenty of those back then, and I'd gotten interest from two: A new TV show in Japan based on the American *Charlie's Angels,* except now with three young women who could dance, sing, act, and host guest stars. There would be one blonde, one brunette, and one redhead, all Caucasian, no Japanese girls. Then, a musical revue with three gals and three guys called *Ski Time* during the ski season, December through the end of March, in Aspen, Colorado. The added perks were free lift tickets for the season and a free place to stay, a large condo for the six cast members.

I had always heard from various sources to be wary of getting hired for shows or modeling jobs in Japan. They were not always on the up and up, and you could really get into a mess there with the job you were hired for being something else entirely, like dancing in a strip club or far worse, a prostitution ring.

Since I had no agent to check this out, I didn't feel it was an option. Back then, once you dropped an agent or they dropped you, that was not kosher. So, I chose the Aspen job.

The show was written by two men, Gene Casey and Hugh Hefner's brother, Keith, who didn't really look like Hef. He was taller and facially very different. He had a cute face, big brown eyes, and was athletic looking. He did have the same voice, and a cute laugh. They were one another's only siblings, and Keith, who was retired, had helped his brother establish all of the Playboy Clubs throughout the U.S. and the world. He had attended Northwestern University in Chicago, where they'd grown up, and received a degree in Drama/Theater Arts. He was an actor in New York and had his own children's TV show for a couple of years, called *Mr. Toby*. But what he'd always loved was Broadway. He had no singing or dancing ability to do that but had the ability to write lyrics to Gene Casey's melodies.

I had just started skiing again a couple of years earlier at Squaw Valley at Tahoe/Donner (and yes, I'm going to call it Squaw, I'm part Native American), and I wanted to get better and do more, which was my main reason for taking the job. I also wanted to sing more, too, and I would have that opportunity, singing solos, trios, and group numbers with some fun songs, along with solo dance parts and comedic sketches. It would be such a good showcase for me.

Ski Time was extremely well written—the jokes and sketches and songs just fit us all like a glove, and the cast got along really well. We had songs like "Rinky Dink Airlines" with two of us as stewardesses and a drunk pilot, "Rocky Mountain Make Out Man", about a gold chain wearing man who trolled the Aspen nightclubs looking for women, and "A Waiting Line", a takeoff on *A Chorus Line*, where I had a dancing and singing solo right out of it, only here, waiting to get on the ski lift instead of getting a Broadway show.

Our costumes were one-piece black ski jumpsuits, and different colored turtleneck shirts. We also were the waiters who served drinks and appetizers, followed by dinner, then performed the first half of the show. We then got off the stage and served after dinner drinks, desserts, and coffee, then got back onstage for the second half of the show. My, oh my, did we have energy or what?

I must go back now to the week of rehearsals, as that is when my relationship with Keith started. We had been working our collective asses off in a ten-day period of time to learn a lot of material, and things were getting tense and grumpy with no days off, so after the Firday rehearsal day ended, Keith called out, "Party at my chalet." We had only been to Mondo Condo, our group condominium, and not to his chalet yet. It was on a private road out of town but not too high up on a hill and it was quite nice, but not really lavish, just comfortable with a small living room, a game room, a basement where the help lived, an upstairs with Keith's bedroom and another spare room, and, of course, a kitchen and dining room.

There was lots of food—pizza, desserts, endless drinks of whatever you wanted—and then there was after dinner vials of cocaine being passed around, also known as "Aspen Snow" because Aspen was famous for an abundance of cocaine, and, of course, it was white. I did not know this until that night, but at least it wasn't freebase!

I hadn't really been attracted to Keith until that night, but I got to sit next to him and get to know him better, and he was simply charming. After about two hours of partying, we were alone in the dining room and we just came together like a scene out of a movie, with a very passionate kiss, about the last thing I expected to happen to me, at least with him.

That night, fireworks went off. I went back to Mondo Condo a short while later, grabbed my overnight case with my flying baby stopper, and went back up to the chalet, and that was that. Of course, we made love, but this time with a twist ... I had my first ORGASM!!!! Sweet mystery of life at last I've found you! Well, he WAS Hugh Hefner's brother, wasn't he? He actually went down on me, yippee and woo hoo! Now I knew that existed, but no man had ever done that to me before, so, finally at age 26, after nine years of having sex, I found out what all the fuss was about. We fell asleep in each other's arms, and the next day I moved out of Mondo Condo and in with Keith.

The next three months were unforgettable, and what a crazy time that was. Except for New Year's Eve, we performed one show a day at 7pm. We'd go skiing most days for half days and then get to Aspen Meadows by 5pm to set up the dining room, change our clothes, and have a lousy employee meal of couscous, with some sort of goulash and vegetables. Our executive chef was the very German, Hans Holzfienz, who had studied at the Cordon Bleu in Paris and was capable of making wonderful cuisine, just not for us. He was also a perfectionist with a temper, and you'd better get that food out when it's up, as he wasn't above throwing plates, food, and utensils, but thank God, no knives!

After the show, I'd go home to Keith, who was sure into the Aspen Snow, as he insisted that we use it every damn night. Then, after my shower, we'd make love or try to, every night, at his suggestion, but as usual with cocaine, he had a hard time with his erection. I was always fine, but then he'd get mad at me for having my climax first.

Still, we were madly in love, and I just learned to deal with it. Once a week on Mondays, the cast and crew took a ski clinic with a very fine instructor, and we learned a tremendous amount. After two weeks, the instructor told me I had to either rent or buy longer skis as I was skiing on 135s, and my own were stiff K2s I had picked up on sale. He said he couldn't teach me any more on my old skis.

I went home and told Keith, and he took me ski shopping the very next day for Rossignol 170s with new bindings and Nordica boots. He also bought me a $500 ski jumpsuit from Paris that was down filled, a light brown color with red lining and a red cap that looked like a jockey's cap. He wanted me to look like a little jockey when we skied together, which was about once a week.

Keith was a beautiful skier like my sister. They both had skied for years, and they were graceful, with close parallel leg positions and turns. Keith had moved to Aspen because of his love of skiing, after he'd finished setting up the final Playboy Club and had become a multi-millionaire. He was just doing *Ski Time* as an entertainment outlet for himself and because there was another successful musical venue downtown, The Crystal Palace, that had good talent and a larger cast of about fifteen singer-dancers. They just performed songs and dances from newer Broadway shows. We went and saw them once, and they were talented young people, but our show was much funnier with our comedic skits and fresh musical score.

We had a parade in January for the annual Winterskol Festival, and it was decided that Keith would rent a flatbed truck and our lead male singer, Danny Nanni, would perform a song that we did nightly, with our three female backup singers behind him. This included me, Jane Holland, and Margaret Taylor singing, "Look at Aspen Now," a takeoff on the 50s song, "Mr. Sandman."

As we made our way down the parade route, people were throwing snowballs at us and yelling all sorts of profanities to be funny. Then someone with a fire hose started spraying people on the floats as they passed by. He didn't hit us, but we screamed and got down on the floor of the flatbed truck anyway. It was scary as the firehose had a lot of force and could have easily knocked us off the truck. Danny and Jane had dropped acid just as the parade had started and were peaking when that happened, and they were so freaked out. I, on the other hand, was sober, and I was freaked out, as well.

This was a Monday, and we had the rest of the day and night off, so we were all invited to Keith's for a party. It's a good thing Keith had help to prepare for all of us. A lot of other various people also came up from the Aspen Meadows, the resort hotel where we performed.

It was a wild, drug fueled scene, as others were on LSD that day as well. They went out in Keith's backyard and literally dragged each other around in the snow. The food, liquor, and vials of cocaine just kept flowing, until everyone eventually went home. Keith and I were finally able to go upstairs, have a jacuzzi, and take a nap.

Keith didn't have that many parties, as the cast usually liked to go into town and troll for significant others at some of the fun bars and nightclubs. Aspen had many hot, attractive young folks and celebrities.

Keith and I were sometimes invited to parties at Aspen millionaires' homes that were incredible. He was considered a local celebrity because he was a Hefner, so the wealthy invited him to brag he had attended their soiree's. We were at a couple of parties with George Hamilton, a tanned Aspen regular, who'd be looking around to see who was looking at him, and Cher, with Greg Allman. Many of these folks were Texas oil millionaires, I later found out.

I'd become a very strong skier. I could ski moguls and black diamonds in a blizzard. All of us became strong skiers because we could ski so often, and of course our tough but superb instructor would stand at the bottom of a mogul run, and yell, "Turn, turn!" and we'd all have to turn instead of procrastinating.

My 27th birthday was March 13th, and *Ski Time* was ending soon, so my birthday party would also be our going away party. The cast bought some weed, and had Hans make me a birthday cake as my gift from them. He sautéed the marijuana and put it into the German chocolate cake batter, so the THC would be effective when we ate the cake. They didn't tell me about it—it was my big surprise.

The cast was so excited, and they could barely wait to sing "Happy Birthday" to me and cut the cake. The cake disappeared in about three minutes flat, and I barely got a piece myself. Then they told me about the secret ingredient—it was too funny! I barely felt the effect, as so many people were handing me vials of cocaine to treat me to a birthday sniff. It was yet another drug fueled Aspen party.

Two weeks later, we said our goodbyes and hoped that the show would run again next winter. It only had two winter runs before ours, and sometimes we had some pretty small audiences. A couple of times, there were as many in the audience as in our cast! We all hoped we'd see each other again for more crazy Aspen times.

Well, now what is next for me and Keith? I'd been letting Alan Creed, a friend of mine, stay at the hut free, as he was finishing chiropractic college in Pasadena. He was leaving now, as I was coming home.

Keith had bought a custom-made Valient sailboat, made in Seattle, and it was in a slip in Marina Del Rey. He'd hardly sailed it yet, so he wanted to come to L.A. and live part time on the sailboat, and part time at his brother's place and/or the Playboy Mansion. He wanted me not to work very much so I could go sailing with him that summer. I could be his crew! Little tiny, skinny me, a one-woman crew for a 40-foot 10-ton sailboat.

That was our basic plan. I had also spoken to my girlfriend Sha about getting an apartment together. She was staying in an older house with a couple of people in the San Fernando Valley, but one was a guy, and I think she just wanted a female roommate for the time being. I wanted a place for my cat, so that's what we did.

We went apartment hunting in the Valley and found a large decent place with two bedrooms and two private bathrooms attached to the rooms, a large living room/dining room with kitchen in between, plus a pool. It had lots of privacy for both of us. I had made a deal with my sister that I would get most of her furniture, as I was paying for storage, so I moved her furniture into my new apartment.

She had come back from Venezuela with a Venezuelan husband and was to pick up her car that my girlfriend Chris was keeping on her street, while we were both gone.

They visited me for a few days before I moved to the new apartment, and my new brother-in-law, Alvaro, was muy loco. He would not leave my sister alone and kept pawing her and she finally had to tell him to stop, and she was crying. I thought, what a mistake, but I didn't want to make it any worse for her. They were driving her beater Toyota to Washington State to see our mom and grandma, and then they were flying to Boca Raton, as Alvaro was going to go to college there.

Sha and I got moved in, the cat got moved in, we are happy, and Keith is coming to town. I saw a dancing audition for a TV special starring Leif Garrett, another teeny bopper pop singer who was only 17, unlike the Bay City Rollers who were in their 20s like me. I always looked a good ten years younger than I was and the call in *Variety* said "Young-looking dancers" so yup, that would be me.

The choreographer was the very nice, very sweet Scott Salmon, with his assistant, Adele Yoshioka. At the call, only four of us were hired, including someone who is still a friend of mine, Denise McKenna. The two other girls were about five years younger than me. There wasn't really much dancing for us to do, and what was given to us was difficult because of the musical interlude we entered on, one at a time, while Leif would dance us up to the stage. When we were all there, the music would change into the John Travolta-inspired "disco point dance" and then we just remained and danced around him.

The song was his smash hit, "I Was Made for Dancing," and I remember telling Leif he was my brother's age, and he looked at me sort of like "Really?" but not bothered. Our costumes were 80s street clothes, and mine was sooo cute, I should've offered to buy it, damn it! Brooke Shields, at sixteen, was his big guest star. I saw her across the soundstage, and her gorgeous eyebrows were noticeable, even from a distance.

CHAPTER TWENTY-SIX

THE PLAYBOY MANSION AND A 40-FOOT 10-TON VALIANT SAILBOAT

Spring 1980, and Keith rolls on in with clothes, mostly, and gets one of the rooms on the second floor of the Mansion. There was the red room, Hef's room, (mostly reserved for celebrity guests like Bill Cosby, a regular) the green, blue, and brown rooms, for family or maybe a Playmate or two of Hef's choosing.

I need the reader to know that what I write about, the activities at the Playboy Mansion are MY TRUTHS, during nine months in 1980.

The Mansion went through many different phases in the 46 years Hef lived there, from 1971 until his death in 2017. There has been a lot written and so much controversy about the goings on, but it was a fluid situation depending on the changing times and popular mores of the times.

For example, when he was still in Chicago at the Playboy Mansion East, there was a lot less debauchery, drugs etc. than the in the mid 70s and for a good decade after that, until Hef re-married and raised children there. During that time, the drugs and group sex came to a halt for a decade. Then it all started up again with his harems of blonde girlfriends for PR purposes, after he and Kimberly Conrad divorced and moved herself and the boys almost next door in Holmby Hills. Later, it finally slowed down to next to nothing in his extreme old age.

It also boggles the mind thinking about his generosity and how many millions of dollars he spent on family, friends, celebrities, Bunnies, Playmates, and others at his parties and events, wining and dining them. When I lived at the mansion with Keith, we could have almost anything we wanted at any time of day, brought to our room by a butler. We ate a lot of fresh cracked crab in drawn butter, our favorite. I will always be grateful to Hugh Hefner for all the great food, and lots of champagne as well!

It worked out so perfectly that I had Sha as a roommate. She was in the very popular Andrew Lloyd Webber musical, *Evita,* as a resident chorus member in the L.A. company, a very steady job. She had a boyfriend, too, and my staying at the Mansion or sometimes on the sailboat afforded her privacy and avoided us getting on each other's nerves. She didn't mind feeding Archie once a day if I wasn't there, but I did come back twice a week for a few hours to give him some love and clean his litter box, so she never had to do that.

After going to the Mansion and meeting Hef, we drove to the sailboat in Marina del Rey, and it was stunning, a sexy sailboat if you will. It had a black hull and a black mast, with a white deck. The name of the boat was the

Renaissance for Keith's re-birth into a life of sailing, and I was happy it made him so happy. The inside of the sailboat had a small but full galley, double bunks, more bunks that were smaller, and a tiny bathroom with a shower. The walls were a reddish-brown wood, and everything was state of the art. Its price tag was $50,000.

Our biggest conundrum was the slip it was in, as it was at the very end of a line of about eight boats in front of us, and it would always be a challenge for us to get it in and out. Our nice neighbors would often come running to help us when we came in, but I was okay being the skinny little 110-pound woman solo crew member on this 10-ton vessel. It's a good thing I grew up on the water, as a professional swimmer and a boater, so I had no fear of the sea. He showed me a few things I'd have to help with, such as fenders out and up, and told me what lines to pull and when. He was confident we could handle the boat by ourselves at least for day sails.

I went back to my apartment, and Sha was there. As we shared a phone and an attached answering machine (no cell phones yet), she told me she'd answered a call from my modeling agent, Joan, and she had a modeling gig for me, and to call her. She had told Sha I'd be playing a young bride and call her asap. I did, and the job was in two days for Mountain Bell Telephone in Colorado, with my favorite photographer, James Wood. Although I told Keith I'd spend the summer sailing with him and not take any major jobs, I was still on call for modeling and TV commercials.

I called Keith and told him I will come over the day after tomorrow on Friday night, after I finish my modeling job to be with him and go to our first Friday night party together. The job was just swell. I was holding a new princess phone that I had just taken out of a gift box, wearing a wedding dress and veil, and my very character typecast husband behind me, looking at a ceramic owl with a look of disgust on his face, as I was holding our gift phone in front of my chest looking soooooo happy. It was a cute print ad.

I got dressed up in my sexy gold tight spandex pants, silk blouse, heels and curled blonde hair, and headed back to Holmby Hills for the weekly Friday night party. I knew how to talk to the rock to let me inside, as I'd been there with Collen, and that had not changed. My name was now on a permanent list. I went up and got Keith, and we both headed downstairs together, Hefner royalty.

It had the same ambiance and feel as before but better now that I was considered family. Clint Eastwood was standing to the right of the staircase by the front door. He was very tall and very thin, borderline gaunt, and we nodded hello to him. A few steps away from him was Kareem Abdul Jabbar, also extremely tall of course, and in front of us on the other side of the foyer was Tony Curtis, looking around bemused. He had the same look the first time I was there, and he seemed to love making eye contact with people, which he did with me. I found out that he was Hef's next door neighbor, and was dating one of the Playmates, Candy Loving. Yes, that was her real name.

We progress to the bar, get our drinks, and go find a table. Lots of guests know Keith, and I am introduced to so many people it makes my head spin. We go through the buffet line and get our dinner and sit back down. What a joy to not have to cook and clean up, always the best part about the Mansion.

We shmooze with some of the older men there, including, agent Lee Wolfberg, Hef's best friend Johnny Dante, Terri Wells, a knockout beauty and who I thought was one of the smarter young women there, and we met Hef's girlfriend, Playmate of the previous year, Sondra Theodore.

Sondra's bedroom was also right next to ours upstairs, so we'd be seeing her a lot. Then, per usual, the movie was shown. We didn't have any interest, so we got another drink, had some "sniffie," and I had my cigarette. Keith had quit smoking a decade ago, but he did tolerate me, as I only smoked maybe six cigarettes a day, and never in the am.

He showed me the playhouse, towards the back of the Mansion grounds, and through the six or so bungalows where the centerfolds stayed when working at the magazine. The game house had several pinball machines, a pool table, and a foosball table, with a bedroom and a bathroom off of it. We went back to the dining room where desserts were being served, but we passed. Keith had his Coca-Cola now and I had a glass of Perrier Jouet champagne, the favorite of all the girls there.

What I did notice is everybody offering everybody else vials of cocaine, palming it to one another, after which they'd disappear into one of several small bathrooms off the foyer and dining area. I had become sick of the drug in Aspen, but Keith was really into it EVERY NIGHT after dinner (at least not before, and with no freebase in sight—thank God for that). And as I got to know some of the other women there, they were very into it as well, that and the Perrier Jouet, as alcohol took the edge off the blow.

I was soon to realize that I'd gone from the Aspen "snow" into the "Playboy blow," the frying pan of drugs into the fire of drugs. It was funny, Hef didn't partake of cocaine or drink much alcohol, but he kept it for his girls. What he did at night was drink Pepsi and smoked weed, while Keith drank Coke and snorted cocaine. Whoever Hef's main squeeze was had to be a superb joint roller. After the movie, Hef would usually go hang out in the game room and Sondra would come in with him and have a flat wooden box and she cleaned the weed of seeds and rolled nice doobies for Hef.

That Sunday, we went back to the sailboat for our first ride. We checked the wind for the day, and it would be enough for a decent sail, and I felt it was now or never. I think that sailing a 40-foot 10-ton sailboat as the solo crew was one of my most noteworthy accomplishments. I was fortunate to be in great shape and have no fear of the water.

It was a gorgeous day, and Keith powered backwards very slowly out of our slip, as I was pulling up the fenders. He then powered us out to sea until we got far enough out of the harbor to be in the open ocean. We headed on out and I helped him pull up the headsail and the mainsail and we were sailing!

Just at that moment, we heard "Ride Like the Wind" by Christopher Cross playing on the radio, and it was like something out of a movie, a perfect soundtrack, so karmic, and I fell in love with the sport. We stayed out for a couple of hours and were one with the sea—no wonder people love it, with the wind and the saltwater air. When we came back, we had to trim both sails on self-rollers and then power up as we reached the harbor and the Marina. We could only go fifteen miles an hour as we went into our slip and again some of the neighbors came running to assist us. What a great day.

We got back in time for Sunday night dinner at the Mansion, which was markedly different than Friday night dinners. Only the closest of family and friends, less drugs, and a much quieter normal ambiance. There was no movie, just the game room, the grotto, and conversation. We were spent after dinner, retired early, made love, and passed out. Sundays were good days there.

It took about two weeks for me to get tired of the Mansion, bigtime. We weren't going to come over to my apartment where there was no free food and beverages, maid and butler service, and cocaine flowing like water, when we could have that at Hef's. Also, I missed my friends and conversing about things other than clothes and cocaine with Hef's girls, as those were their main points of interest.

Two great events were an honorary banquet and award party thrown by the city of Hollywood honoring Hef's philanthropy to the City of Hollywood, and an awards banquet for Francis Albert Sinatra that Hef threw at the Mansion. I had no gown for either, so Keith sent me shopping in Beverly Hills for a gown and heels that I would use for both. I chose a white Grecian gown, cocktail-length, and a pair of copper-silver heels that tied around my ankles.

The first event was tied to Hef getting his star on the Hollywood Walk of Fame in April, but this was the actual Humanitarian Banquet Award thrown by the City of Hollywood for his help saving the Hollywood Sign. Hef and Keith's mother Grace, and Hef's daughter Christy flew in from Chicago, as it was a substantial honor for Hef.

So Hef and Sondra, Keith and I, Christy and Grace pile into the white stretch limo, and head on into Hollywood to the Palladium Ballroom. As we pull up, the paparazzi was ready and waiting for us, and there are about a dozen fans with photos for Hef to sign. The limo driver protects us as best he can, but the paparazzi even want to know my name and if I'm Hef's girlfriend. I shake my head no. It's a wild scene.

Inside is formal, quiet and serene, with white table cloths, champagne, and then dinner. Debbie Reynolds does her one-woman show in his honor and jeeze was it good. She could do celebrity impressions that were so real it made your jaw drop, and of course, she sang "Tammy" and a few other songs. She was very entertaining. Hef then got up and gave a speech thanking everyone, and then we left with no paparazzi, nice and peaceful.

A couple of weeks later, Hef hosted the big black tie party honoring Frank Sinatra, with a full orchestra and dancing, a banquet, and all the booze one could drink.

So, same Grecian gown and heels, and afterwards lots of booze and blow, and no, I didn't get to actually meet Francis Albert, but I could see his blue eyes.

Paranoia strikes deep. Back in Aspen, Keith had already started in with the cocaine paranoia and temper that goes along with a lot of cocaine usage. He knew of my last two relationships with long haired hippie-rockers. I could hardly hide those, they were public domain, and of course, men closer to my age.

Once, when we were at the Paragon night spot in Aspen with the cast, listening to fun, live dance music, he would not dance with me, so Chris, our young long-haired piano player asked me to dance with him and boy did I catch hell afterwards, even though Keith wouldn't dance me! It was stupid, because Chris was gay and we all knew that! So, I had to be careful of any conversation or interaction with younger, longer haired men when Keith was around.

When I saw Robin Williams standing all by himself a few weeks later at a Friday night party I said to Keith, "Look, look, there's Robin Williams all by himself! Let's go and talk to Mork from the planet Ork!" and he was on board with that! Robin was so friendly as we introduced ourselves, and we were so happy to hang out with him. One thing I noticed after about ten minutes is that Robin was ON ALL THE TIME, cracking jokes with his whip smart mind. I was like "Knock knock, where's the real Robin?" But he was just so congenial, so adorable!

The next week at the Friday party Robin was there again with his first wife, Valerie, who was a modern dancer he met at Juilliard. She was on the plain side unlike most of the rest of the women there. We were in the game room after dinner, and we just talked to Robin a little bit, and Valerie looked fairly unhappy to be in that setting.

Also, that same night, hanging in the game room was Carrie Fisher with Monty Python's Eric Idle. Carrie looked pretty unhappy as well. Carrie and Valerie looked like I felt being there! I went over to her and introduced myself as one of the Wookies in the Star Wars TV special and told her that I was at her mom's dance studio a lot as I was a dancer/singer rehearsing there, and how much I appreciated Debbie's studio. She made no eye contact with me and said something like, "I don't talk to my mom," and I said, "Well okay," and moved away.

Then the next Friday, Robin was by himself again, and Keith and I gravitated over to him, and he seemed happy to be with us. I had asked Keith when I saw Robin if I could ask him and his wife to come sailing with us that Sunday, and Keith said okay, so I did. Robin politely declined as he had a gig for the next week at the Comedy Store on Sunset Strip, but he asked us to come and be his guests three nights later, and he'd comp us in. So of course, we said yes, and we went as Robin's guests.

What an enlightening experience that was, at least for me. He surely was not Mork from the planet Ork, he was a sexual, dirty, F-bomb stand-up, just a tad less dirty than Richard Pryor had been in concert. I enjoyed it because it was Robin but was shocked by his change of material. We waited after the show in the lobby to see him, thank him, and tell him how much we enjoyed him, and that was the last we ever saw of him, at the Mansion at least, and I will never forget him. He started doing films, and the rest is history. I'm sure he is making God laugh in heaven.

Keith wanted me to learn to play tennis as he was a superb tennis player and even played in celebrity tennis tournaments from time to time, as he was considered a minor celebrity.

I played some tennis, but it was not a good choice for me. It involved running on asphalt courts, and it gave me shin splints, bad for my dance career. Plus, I simply didn't like it as much as I enjoyed skiing, swimming, horseback riding, sailing, or even just watching competitive sports. But I was trying to do something Keith wanted me to do with him more. I had a little baby tennis racket, a tennis outfit that I used for print work and commercial auditions, and tennis shoes, of course.

We decided the next day we'd go down to the court and practice some tennis, as the Mansion had a nice tennis court. I woke up before Keith the next morning, had some coffee and a croissant, and headed on down to the court with some balls to practice before Keith came down, but there was somebody else practicing. His name was Bill Cosby.

Of course, I knew who he was, and I knew he stayed there often but he was never at any parties, not even Sunday family-style parties. Nope, he was like a ghost guest. I said hi and told him I just wanted to practice my serve. He said, "Go ahead, I'll watch you," which he did, and then started to give me some pointers on what to do. This went on for about five minutes, before Keith arrived.

Of course, Keith and Bill knew one another, and Bill just stuck around and watched Keith and I try to play some tennis—what a joke! Keith got impatient with me after about two serves and Bill tried to give me advice, as he saw and heard that Keith could not tolerate my inept ability with a racket. It all only lasted about another ten minutes before Keith and I called it quits, but of course it was a memorable experience.

Much later in life, I found out from my modeling agent Joan Mangum, that she would never send any of us young women on any audition with Bill, as he was a well-known sexual harasser and sometimes worse. I was so grateful to her for that. She said every agent in Hollywood knew he was a bad man when it came to young women, and they'd send their gals anyway to make a buck! I never encountered him again at the Mansion or anywhere else. I had guardian angels, I swear, and one was Joan Mangum.

July 4th at the Mansion was one of Hef's disco roller-skating parties that were fun to watch and were well attended. He'd turn the tennis court into a roller rink, rent a bunch of roller skates, and mostly Playmates, Bunnies, and celebrities took part.

I hadn't skated in years, so I didn't feel confident to participate. The next day was the Playboy Jazz Festival, and lots of us went with Hef and Sondra and Terri Wells, in a group of limos. I was able to invite my BFF, Bridget, to accompany Hef's friend, Lee Wolfberg, and we all got pink satin jackets commemorating the 25th anniversary of the magazine. It was late afternoon, and we saw the band Hiroshima and others, and then we went back to the Mansion for more champagne and cocaine.

July meant sailing on Sundays, mostly, and during the rest of the week, I'd go home for a day, take a dance class or two, and then go back to the Mansion.

Keith's temper and behavior towards me was becoming more and more belittling and paranoid. He got down on me for not watching more news, about two hours nightly at dinnertime, and if I said I admired an iconic female figure like Katharine Hepburn or Meryl Streep, he'd yell at me and say, "Then be more like them." He also drank two very dry martinis with dinner every night before he switched to Coke and cocaine and his temper would flare badly at martini time. Gin drinkers, you know?

One night it was particularly bad. He was so verbally abusive it brought me to tears. I got in my Z and drove home to the Valley to kitty and Sha. Also, Hef had asked Keith if we would like to join the Friday night orgy in his room, a group of about eight to ten men and women with him, Terri Wells, Sondra Theodore, a couple more Playmates and a couple more of his male friends on Hef's huge bed.

Usually, Sondra was the wrangler for this, but because Keith was Hef's brother, Hef asked us himself. Keith had come to me and asked if I would like that, and I said, "Please, no." I mean, my God, I'd left Al two years ago because of orgy participation, and here's more orgies! Keith also didn't like group sex, so he was fine with my decision as well. It just seemed like all of Los Angles was rampant with orgies and blow in the late 70s/early 80s.

I needed to get away from the Mansion, or at least not spend so much time there. Keith called me at my apartment and apologized and told me how much he loved me and how much our relationship meant to him and asked me to come back. I said yes, as long as we lived on the sailboat more and not the Mansion, and he said yes, and we did! It was the most peaceful month of our relationship, by far. We did no cocaine, and we even sailed to Catalina Island. It was so idyllic.

Keith also booked a theatre trip to NYC for us to see Broadway shows, the first week of September. It was so exciting.

Earlier, on August 14th, there had been the Dorothy Stratten tragedy that was just so horrible. The Mansion should've been draped in black, as the few times we went back later that month, the grief was just palpable, as she was very loved by all who knew her.

CHAPTER TWENTY-SEVEN

THE BEST AUDITION OF MY LIFE, THE MR. BLACKWELL GIRL

Everybody knew who Mr. Blackwell was in the 70s. He was so visible on TV all the time on many talk shows. He'd been a highly successful women's clothing designer in the 60s, upscale expensive ladies' gowns, and the like. In the late 70s he'd become a fashion critic and had the top ten list of the worst dressed celebrity women and men. When he came out with the worst dressed list every year, I looked forward to it because his descriptions of the stars' wardrobe choices were acerbic, hilariously delivered in a snobby yet devilishly smiling manner on TV that was quite enjoyable.

My commercial agent called me with an audition for a new hair care line under the Mr. Blackwell name. He was searching for a good-looking young woman, with beautiful hair, in her 20s, who could do nonverbal acting, and who could dance. I'd always wanted to represent hair care or shampoo as I did have beautiful hair, and my eyes were my best feature. So, I was mildly excited, although I thought my competition would be fierce—ya know, like more Farrah Fawcett, but she already represented Wella Balsam, a conflict of interest, ha ha!

I went back to the apartment and prettied up, got my Zed card and resumé and went to the audition, enthusiastically hopeful. It was in an ornate building, inside a large room with a high ceiling, and a large open door with a sign that read: "Mr. Blackwell Audition Here."

I walked through the door and Mr. Blackwell was talking to some people. As I got closer, he turned and looked at me and said to no one in particular, "That's it, there she is, shut the call down."

I didn't think he meant me. I looked behind me, but nobody was there, so it was me!!! I had my headshot, Zed, and resumé visibly in hand and I said, "Don't you even want to see this?" with a big smile. "You can dance, right?" was his reply. "You are perfect, just what I envisioned."

He looked at the info. "Linda, I'm Richard, it's my new hair care line. It will pay SAG regional scale with an option to go National, and we'll shoot around the first to the third of September in Solvang, an overnight shoot all expenses covered. We'll drive you, and please call me Richard," all said with his devilish smile. He continued, "This is my costumer, let her take your measurements, and you are done. I'll call your agent, and we'll let you know the exact shoot date when we know. Thank you for being here and see you again soon."

Still in a state of shock, I had my measurements taken and left. Was this a dream? NO, it was reality and just fantastic. Why can't all auditions be like this? I did not go home. I went to the Mansion where Keith and I were staying that night for the first time in a while. I was bursting with joy and excitement to tell him!

I did tell Keith, almost screaming with excitement, and a very dark cloud came over his face. "Do you realize what this coincides with?" he said. "Our New York theater trip on September 1st. I bought tickets for both of us to see five Broadway shows, with reservations at the Essex House, and airline tickets as well. I cannot change the show tickets this late and that's $1,000 lost. You are going to have to tell Mr. Blackwell you cannot do the shoot." He was trying to control himself as best he could.

Tears filled my eyes, and I asked if we could just change the tickets to a later date but again the answer was no. So, I got my agent on the phone and explained the painful situation to her, and she said she'd talk to Mr. Blackwell, personally. I sat there shattered, heartbroken on so many levels. The phone rang about twenty minutes later. It was Richard Blackwell himself wanting to speak to me, as Keith had answered our room phone.

"Hi Linda, it's Richard and your agent explained the situation to me. You know what? I'll wait for you to get back, not that long, right?"

I double checked our dates with Keith who was right there and said yes. He said, "Fine, we can wait for you, but we'll go to Solvang probably the day after you return so don't party too hard. Enjoy your shows, I love Broadway."

"Thank you, thank you, thank you," I said ecstatically. "I really want to be your hair care girl for your product. I'm so grateful and honored." That had never happened either, unbelievable! Broadway here we come!

What a great trip. We saw *A Day in Hollywood, A Night in the Ukraine*, the revival of *Camelot* with Richard Burton and Christine Ebersole from the 4th row, incredible, although Richard Burton was very stiff in his body movements,

Barnum (my least favorite), *Little Shop of Horrors* off-Broadway with Ellen Greene, and the opulent *42nd St.* That was important for me to see as I would be up for a part in it in a couple of years.

We dined at some of the finest restaurants Manhattan had to offer: Tavern on the Green, The Russian Tea Room (my personal favorite), and 21, where we saw Frank Sinatra holding court just three tables away. Keith was in heaven, but he didn't bug him.

We also went to a rooftop party thrown by my alumni and director of my stage production of *Grease,* Dan O'Conner, and our *Ski Time* castmate Jane Holland was there as she now lived in NYC.

On the final day I took Carol Lugenbeal to Café des Artistes for lunch without Keith as he had drunk too much at the rooftop party and wanted to sleep it off, but he treated us. Then, we went back to Carol's small apartment and smoked a doobie, and I barely made it back to the Essex House. All in all, a fantastic trip and NO COCAINE. Keith couldn't carry a schedule two narcotic on a plane! Ha ha!!!

We get back to L.A. and Keith has the limo drop me at home because I must repack and go to Solvang tomorrow and shoot my Mr. Blackwell Hair Care commercial.

The next morning, a van picks me up with the director, stylist, and cameraman, and we head north about two hours and twenty minutes. The stylist shows me the dress she has for me: A light chiffon dress with a floral print, ruffled off the shoulder with spaghetti straps for support, feminine and lovely.

We go to our hotel. Solvang is beautiful, a quaint Danish village but with a windmill. Richard is there in the lobby already dressed in a suit, and he greets us. We go to our assigned rooms to unpack, and I have to get into my pretty dress. I go back down to the lobby, and our stylist is putting Richard's makeup on and his hair, and then mine.

The director talks to me about the shots and what I will do: Dancing down the main street, happily doing chassés with flowing ballet arms to some pleasant non-descript background music, then stopping to look in a pastry shop with the camera shooting me from the inside, then a chaînés turn into Mr. Blackwell's outstretched arm, and I put my hand on his shoulder and look at him adoringly. He has been doing a voiceover talking about his products as I perform this thirty-second ad.

We do takes all day, then we all go to dinner with the Danish partners of the hair care line, which was the reason we are in Solvang, and why I was chosen for my Scandinavian looks, and blonde locks.

We head back to L.A. mid-morning, and everyone is happy, and I'm told by Richard he would call me when it starts running. I was given several bottles of shampoo and conditioner, which I used and really enjoyed. But as time goes by, I do not hear from him??? HMMMM?

Years later, up in Seattle when I moved back, I went to a book signing of his life story titled *From Rags to Bitches*, and he recognizes me despite my shorter hair and some weight gain. I asked him what happened with the hair care line and our commercial. "The Danish people ran away with my money and the product, back to Denmark, so it was never sold here," was his sad reply, and I was sad for us both. But I bought his book, and he signed it, fondly, to me, and at least I got to see him again. He may have been feared by some folks, but he was nothing but a teddy bear to me.

CHAPTER TWENTY-EIGHT
VIVA LAS VEGAS

It's getting on to the end of September now, and I'm running out of money. I really haven't worked much over the summer, and soon I'll be out of unemployment as well. Also, Keith found out that the Aspen Meadows resort will no longer present *Ski Time* for a third Winter, as it didn't make enough money the past two to make it worth their while. I needed a job that would make me some money that I could live on. It will soon be too cold to take the sailboat out, and Keith will probably go back to Aspen for ski season, as it IS his home.

I saw an ad in *Variety* that said female dancers needed who can sing and act, no height requirement, for a lounge show, a 50s musical revue for Dick Clark Productions. It was *Dick Clark's Nifty 50s Revue*, playing Las Vegas for six weeks.

Well, I just did a revue, and I liked the format, so I auditioned and got the job, and it did more than earn me money, it got me away from the Mansion and cocaine. I don't care what Keith says or how mad he gets—he doesn't want to support me, so he cannot say no.

The show will run through December 8th, 1980, and then we can go to Aspen for the holidays. But he didn't get upset, and I started rehearsals in L.A. for a few days, and then we progressed to Vegas.

We were playing in the lounge at the Marina Hotel, a smaller hotel that had about fifteen floors, a casino, and our lounge showroom. If you were never in Vegas in the 70s and 80s, it was very different than it is now. There were much fewer hotels and casinos, and not all that much to do, not like the Disneyland it would become.

The show ran just under an hour. We were six cute gals, all of us no taller than 5'5", and we did most of our dancing in poodle skirts, ponytails, full shirts with cap sleeves, and Capezio heels. The song "Itsy Bitsy Teeny Weeny Yellow Polka Dot Bikini" featured us in very conservative bikinis that were under our poodle skirt costume. Four of us changed into these behind a beach towel held up by the other two girls. We were known as the most clothed show in Vegas at that time.

Our choreographer was the very funny, very swishy Jerry Grimes, who created some fast and entertaining choreography for the six of us.

The stars of the show were Danny and the Juniors from the 1950s, whose hit song was "Dancing at the Hop" that we ponied around the stage to, while they sang. We opened the show with a version of "American Bandstand." We had a comedian, Carl Waxman, who would make fun of the six of us standing around the stage behind him, and then he also did about ten minutes of stand-up on his own.

On opening night, Dick Clark showed up to introduce us, with the press in attendance, and I got my picture in a Vegas paper, singing, microphone in hand. I made friends with some of the girls, including Dani Douthette, who is still my friend. I also had friends coming from L.A. to see me.

We were put up in a cheap hotel, attached to the Marina by a breezeway. The rooms were provided for us, and we also got a discount at the adjacent coffee shop. Keith came to visit me twice and got us a room at Caesars, the best place in Vegas at the time. We had some fun times with other cast members and their boyfriends, dining after the show.

In early November, my modeling agent had a job for me at a Union 76 station outside of L.A. close to the Ontario airport, just east of LAX. She knew that I was in Vegas, but she asked me anyway and I told her I'd talk to my boyfriend about it, as it would be on the first Monday of November, a dark day off for me. The next day is voting day, and I am a registered California voter. Keith's mind was moving fast, so he said, "I'll fly you in, and the next morning we'll go and vote and then you can fly back early in time to do your Tuesday night show."

Keith and Hef were really concerned about the 1980 election for president, as Ronald Reagan was threatening to crack down on porn, and that meant Playboy. So, I did the print job for Union 76, behind the counter of a real Union 76 station, and received my hourly rate of $110. Keith picked me up and we went back to the Mansion, and we stayed clean, no cocaine.

The next morning, we got up and exercised our right to vote. I am instructed and expected to vote for Jimmy Carter, but I have not been impressed with his four years in office, so I tell Keith OF COURSE, whatever you want dear, and I get in that booth, draw the curtain, and vote for the stronger man, Ronald Reagan. I will always love Jimmy Carter as a sublime human being, just not as a world leader. At the time, I didn't even know that my stepdad, Harold Michael, was a secret service man for the Gipper at the Santa Barbara ranch. Finally, I flew back to Vegas, $110 richer.

The other cast members got to see Ann Margret's show, as she had a different dark night. I was bummed I missed it. You could go to see other people's shows at that time for free if you had a night off. My chiropractor friend, Dr. Alan Creed came to the rescue for me. He was treating Ann-Margret's two backup singers, and they invited him to come to Vegas and to a party that Roger Smith was throwing for her after both of our shows one night. He took me! It was in the Presidential Suite at Caesars, and it had a hot tub, so I was told to bring my bathing suit.

We walked in and there she was, my beautiful role model that I'd waited all of my life to meet, and what happened??? I was tongue-tied. The boy dancers had made an arm swing for her, and she was sitting in it, so happy, as two of them swung her back and forth. I really could not speak or introduce myself, but sort of stared at her in awe. So, we had some food from the buffet table, took a hot tub with the backup singers and left. I blew that opportunity to thank her, but at least I got to be close to her.

Monday, December 8th was our last night, and we had to do one last show to fulfill our contract. We had packed up our cars, ready for the modest five-hour drive across the desert back to L.A. It was a hilarious show, and we just goofed off the entire time and laughed our asses off. There were only about ten people in the audience, including our one hotel hooker, that our show manager let in free, and the wait staff, etc.

My friend, Andi Cappola got onstage with a bucket hat on, and did her imitation of "Gene Gene, the Dancin'

Machine" from *The Gong Show*, and we threw a roll of toilet paper all over comic Carl Waxman's head. About two-thirds of the way through the show, someone from the hotel staff came to us backstage and told us John Lennon had been gunned down and killed in front of his apartment building, the Dakota, in New York. We were in a state of shock for the remainder of our show and the lead singer of Danny and the Juniors held a moment of silence for him at the end of the show.

We said our goodbyes, and Andi and I drove through the night, listening to continual John Lennon and Beatles songs on my car radio as the sun came up over L. A. We wept on and off for the five-hour drive, a tragedy that marked my one Vegas show.

It was Christmastime and time to go back to Aspen with Keith. I put on my lynx-dyed fox fur, "Chubbie," that Keith had bought me right before we went to New York, and my real Aspen Stetson hat, two Aspen essentials for the elite crowd.

Sondra Theodore had sort of scolded Keith for not buying me a fur coat, so he took me to Beverly Hills Furrier and purchased my $2,500 jacket, as all of the Hefner brother's women should have at least one. It was a status symbol back then, a BIG no-no now. I was trying not to cry as I really didn't want to go back to Aspen for the holidays because I knew what it would entail.

There was a lack of snow in Aspen that winter, which happens from time to time, yet another reason Aspen Meadows didn't want our show back, a lack of tourists. Keith's good friend Les Irons had opened a gift shop in the Aspen Mall downtown, which had flourished last season, but was bankrupt now, once again from lack of tourists. That is the precarious part of choosing to have a retail business in any town that depends on snow to survive. Keith had put money into it to help him, but now all was lost, and Les was also having to stay downstairs in a spare room, as he had no money. They both sat around, very depressed.

I went skiing by myself only twice, as the slopes were partially bare, with some rocks exposed, and Keith didn't want to ruin his skis. Of course, there was the usual use of sniffie, but towards the end of the three weeks, I was hardly doing any.

We did have a nice New Year's Eve with plenty of Veuve Clicquot, my favorite French champagne. We had what I thought was a decent tête-à-tête about cocaine use and how I wanted both of us to stop using it. I felt it would help our relationship, and asked could we please work on that? He said yes, but I needed to go back to L.A. and take care of Archie and look for work, which I did, the entire month of January.

The next time I came back, a few days before Valentine's Day, not much had transpired in the way of Keith cutting back on cocaine. He even suggested that we start dropping acid from time to time, which I had not done in almost eight years, and I said, "No, I could cause more damage to my chromosomes, especially with my previous drug usage, and I may want children in the future. NOOOOOO!

I'd been there about three days, when one morning I got up first and I went downstairs, approaching the kitchen, when I heard the housekeeper/chef and Les talking about the week before when Debby was there—hmmm—when Debby was there? I came around the corner and I asked, "Who's Debby?" They both looked like they'd seen a ghost. Les spoke first and said, "Well I guess Keith hasn't told you, but he's also been seeing an old girlfriend who left her husband. I'm sure he was going to talk to you about it. We're sorry you heard us talking about her, we did not mean to spill the beans."

I knew who they were talking about immediately. Keith had shown me a picture of her from a while back and she was a knockout! HUGE blue eyes and a brunette, such a beautiful combination with milky white skin, and lovely face. He had told me she had left him to marry a televangelist, and that she was a religious nutball. That cracked me up!

Keith came down, and after breakfast I mentioned what had transpired and told him it was not his friend or the help's fault, but I'd found out he was seeing Debby. The last time we spoke, I believe we'd agreed he'd work at stopping cocaine use, so we could have a better relationship. He blew up and said he was not going to quit using it, he liked the drug too much, and Debby would allow him to keep using it. A HUGE fight ensued fueled by more blow, and I made arrangements to fly home early the next day, taking my Rossignol's with me.

Some of you may be wondering why it took me this long to break it off. Well, I was in love with him, and he also had a sexual hold on me. He WAS charming and he had a fun personality. After all, he was entertaining enough to have a children's television show in New York. I saw him one last time when I picked up my deep-sea fishing pole he'd bought for me while sailing. I'd caught many mackerel with it (catch and release), as I still enjoyed fishing from my youth. He was pleasant and seemed to be happy with his choice of Debby, and it was all for the best for me.

If you want to read another book or excerpt from it, Debby Keener has written a book about their marriage, life after the birth of their disabled daughter, and subsequent divorce, entitled, *Don't Panic*. She did me a big favor by taking Keith out of my life, and that book is her truth.

It took a while to get him out of my heart. I found myself only looking at men fifty or older for about six months afterwards but not acting on it.

And for those of you wanting more stories about the Playboy Mansion in the late 70s and early 80s, there's nothing quite as revealing and courageous as Sondra Theodore's true account documentary, *Secrets of Playboy,* that premiered in 2022. It contains interviews with many more Playmates and girlfriends of Hugh Marston Hefner, and his second-floor goings on, as I called them. If you just went to the parties at various time periods over the years, it was a fluid situation that could change, depending on Hef's wants and needs. But I was LIVING on the second floor and experienced a lot more than the vast majority of people who simply visited the Mansion and were never invited upstairs.

Sondra and the others were telling their TRUTH, as I am telling mine, and Debby Keener, hers. I never went to the Mansion again and never did cocaine again. Good riddance to both.

CHAPTER TWENTY-NINE

FREE AT LAST

After the previous three relationships, I was done for quite a while. Oh sure, I dated, but I would not have any substantial chemistry now with anyone for several years to come. I wasn't looking for marriage yet, and still had some unfinished career goals to accomplish, like working on Broadway.

How refreshing to be back in my own apartment, with my own friends and true contemporaries, who were drug free for the most part. About the worst thing we did was drink wine, margaritas, and on wild occasions, tequila shooters, but most certainly not on a daily basis. We also smoked cigarettes, Virginia Slims to be exact, but my limit was two cigarettes a day, and never before noon.

I did a print job for Joan Mangum for a steel company in the seat of a roller coaster, as a sort of floozie young woman on a date with her sailor boyfriend. It was cute, easy, and rather obscure work, and I found it enjoyable. I was auditioning for a few things here and there but trying not to go back to just dancing for a while. I really enjoyed putting all three talents to good use or just taking acting or modeling jobs.

We had a couple of pool parties at our Kling Street apartment with our friends and some of the *Evita* cast. Sha threw an *Evita* girls chorus slumber party with PJs and sleeping bags—that was really unique for women in their 20s. I was the token non-*Evita* member. Sha's then boyfriend, Steve Canyon Kennedy, and his friend Scott Holmes would come over and hang with us occasionally in the daytime before evening *Evita* performances.

Scott was the star of *Evita*, playing at the Shubert Theater in Century City. When Keith and I were still together, we went to see it, and there was Scott as Che Guevara. What a role and what a talent. Scott was devilishly handsome with almost jet-black hair, blue eyes, a perfect nose almost like mine (I did have a good one), and a pirate's smile. Also, a wonderful sense of salty humor, like mine. There was an instant attraction for both of us, and a lot of chemistry, but there was this little problem in the way called marriage.

Scott was married to a lovely, pretty woman, Pamela, a stewardess. As I mentioned, Scott would come over and hang out with us sometimes. We had some physical interaction, but I was not going to be a homewrecker (bad karma). After all, she was also his college sweetheart, so we just became friends, buddies, and talked on the phone from time to time.

My 28th birthday came around in March, and Sha made me a cake and invited my friends over to a morning birthday get-together for toast, coffee and cake. It was cute and just right for me.

Recently, I'd been talking to Al Kooper. We were slowly becoming friends again, and Sha invited him. Al had hooked up with a blue-eyed blonde graphic artist, Patti Heid, who moved into a rental house with him after he had to sell Freebird Mansion. She was attractive but not in showbiz, so not really glamorous. They had moved to England for a while and were with George Harrison at his country mansion the day John Lennon got gunned down at the Dakota. Al was doing some session work for George. It was a dark time for all of us, but particularly the other Beatles.

They then moved to Austin, as it had a thriving music scene, and I think Al was hoping to find a new band there that he could produce and have another Lynyrd Skynyrd-type success, but that just didn't happen. He and Patti did hang with my friend, Bremerton songwriter-musician-singer Bill Carter for a while, as Bill was the epicenter of the Austin music scene, and the who's who of all things rock and pop music there, but they never really collaborated.

Patti had had enough of Al, and they split up, and now they were both back in L.A. Patti had somehow met Cheech Marin of Cheech and Chong, and they had just gotten married! Al was alone again, and probably on the orgy circuit again, but I certainly wasn't interested, although I did like being friends with him.

April came around and I had to start aggressively looking for a job now, although I was still floating on unemployment and my meager savings, taking dance classes and hanging out with the Los Angles cast of *Evita*, now in its second year. It was just that good and that popular.

Since I've got a slight lapse here in my story until the next job, I'm going to go back to June of 1980 at the Playboy Mansion. Sha relayed to me that I had a work call from an

Alan Johnson, a choreographer, on the message machine, and a phone number to call him back asap.

I had never worked for him, but I knew of his name as a working choreographer in L.A. I called him back and he introduced himself as the choreographer for Mel Brooks' new comedy *A History of the World Part 1.* He had gotten my name from one of the other women he was working with. He was responsible for a synchronized swim routine and scene in Mel's movie. She had told him that I was a capable synchronized swimmer.

I would not have to audition, just show up for rehearsals and filming. It was five days—two rehearsal days and three filming days—for $1,000 and guaranteed residuals. I said sure—I loved Mel Brooks, oh boy! I would be a swimming nun in the Spanish Inquisition scene and do a little simple dancing as well.

I go from a tap-dancing vagina and a teenage Wookie to a swimming nun. That's entertainment, right? I arrive on set for the first day of rehearsal, and the soundstage is huge and amazingly decked out with our elevated pool, with two narrow platforms on the right and left sides, various devices of torture on a large platform behind the pool, and a slide coming down into the pool from the back.

There was a stage below the pool from right to left, more long than wide but a decent-sized area, big enough for Torquemada and his dancing monks. This was Stage 32 at Paramount which Howard Hughes had built for parties.

I don't know how much y'all know about the hideous Spanish Inquisition, but it goes something like this: Spain was trying to rid itself of all Jews and Muslims and become a completely Catholic country. The King and Queen of Spain had put the cleanse in the hands of a Dominican friar, Tomás de Torquemada, to ferret out, torture and kill those Jews and Muslims who would not give up everything they owned to the Spanish government and move to another country—with the help of the Spanish army of course. He was famous for torturing and killing into the thousands of Jews in our scene, while many thousands of others were burned at the stake as heretics.

Mel Brooks is portraying Torquemada, a dancing and singing Grand Inquisitor who, with his monks and nuns, are in progress of doing just that: torturing and killing Jews in a fun loving, joyful manner, with synchronized swimming, and song and dance! Mel is trying everything he can with his torture devices to get the Hasidic Jews to confess to I don't know what, but they won't speak, so he says, "Bring in the nuns," and the sixteen of us enter from the stage left platform with robes on and white swim caps, in prayer, with our heads bowed.

We spread out to a straight line on the edge of the pool, simultaneously open and drop our robes behind us, to expose white bathing suits, turn to the front with arms in dive position over our heads, and do a side peel off dive one by one, like dominoes, into the pool below. The camera then cuts to us doing synchronized front strokes in four lines of four across the pool, and then to under water shots of back dolphins (I'm in the front), followed by some of the Jews coming down the slide to us. The next scene, which was cut from the film, was with Mel, off camera, counting down, "3,2,1," as the nuns in a corner of the pool, squealed "Jews." We then pull them under the water and drown them with a bubble that comes up that say, "Oy!" Finally, a spinning menorah comes out of the water, with eight nuns instead of Hannukah candles, as Mel and his monks sing and dance "The Inquisition."

It was sheer Mel genius.

Three of the monks were my fellow dancers or choreographers: Jimmy Roddy, Dom Salinaro, and Stan Mazin, who was my partner on *The Carol Burnett Show*. He got to speak a line to Mel Brooks! It made it more fun for the monks to be with us. The funny thing to this day is that none of my other girlfriends on the job, about five of them, remembers who the swim choreographer was. We were not the swim choreographers, and Alan Johnson and Charlene Painter, his very sweet assistant, just stood by the side of the pool and watched us. They knew nothing about synchronized swimming. Alan was always Mel Brooks' choreographer for all his movies. He choreographed the monks and Mel, and our step kicks at the finale.

The movie came out in June of 1981 and was a HUGE hit for dear Mel. It has made me about $20,000 over the past forty-five years. I still get residuals to this day, and you can often stream it for free if you've never seen it. I'm third nun from the end on the side peel off dive!!!

Hef and I did have a conversation about both of us working on *History of the World Part 1* in June of '80. Hef had shot the Roman Empire scene before me, and I was in the Spanish Inquisition scene after him. Mel hired him to walk around the streets of Rome with some of his recent Playmates in Roman togas, playing themselves. I told him what I was doing, and we both had a good laugh about the history aspect. We couldn't wait to see the finished product

Back to 1981 and it's May. I auditioned for *Evita* but aww c'mon, I was just too blonde to play an Argentinian commoner—only Eva Perón could be blonde. And then, as my good fortune and karma would have it, I get a call from Jerry Jackson, my previous choreographer from the company of *Seven Brides for Seven Brothers*, that I had done almost three years ago with Jane Powell and Howard Keel. He told me that *Seven for Seven* was being re-mounted again, this time with pop singing star Debby Boone. I could have my bride role back. I would not have to audition (this did happen with fair frequency more than I thought at the beginning of this memoir) but to please come to the open call audition and meet my producers Larry Kasha and

David Landay. I could sit at the audition table and observe, but the part was mine if I wanted it.

Oh, hell yes, and it would be a tour of another Kenley Circuit, but this one was the Midwest: Akron, Columbus, and Dayton, and finishing up in Flint, Michigan. The tour would start at the end of May and go through the first week in August. It was principal pay with per diem, and then hopefully in the Fall, rehearsing in L.A. with possibly a partial new cast, a national tour, then on to Broadway! I would originate my principal bride role on Broadway!!!

I went to the open call audition and met Larry Kasha and David Landay, partners in business and partners in real life as well. They were very nice and were happy I'd said yes. Craig Peralta was also there—he'd had played Gideon, the ethereal tenor who was the star behind Debby and whomever her Adam would turn out to be.

Debby was not there, I would meet her later, but Craig's new bride partner Nancy Fox was there—she'd be replacing Dorothy Nichols per Craig's request.

Apparently, there had been yet an earlier tour with Jane and Howard that I was not aware of that Nancy had done with Craig of *Seven for Seven* and Craig had become close friends with her and liked working with her, but not romantically. I had done *Hello, Dolly!* at Sacramento Music Circus with Nancy as Minnie Fay, and she was a VERY cute, very good comedic actress. What a feeling of power to sit behind the audition table and not hopping and sweating in front of it. It was interesting to see others stressed out trying to get a job, just the vibe. They chose some to stay for a callback, but they were going to NYC to audition hopefuls there, so we would see the final full cast when in Akron.

Akron was the home of the Goodyear Tire Company, and you could tell the minute you got to the place—the entire city smelled like rubber tires ALL THE TIME. I don't know about you, but I HATE the smell of tires, and now I have to live with it for three weeks. Actually, once you went inside, the smell abated.

I was first taken to my semi-shitty motel room that I would be sharing with Debby Boone's understudy, Terri Homberg, who I barely knew. She was a pleasant but very hyper young woman, with lots of nervous energy. She was dating my fellow classmate, D. Scott Davidge, who was playing second to the oldest Pontipee brother Benjamin.

About an hour after we get settled, I hear a knock at my door, and it is my dance partner, Michael Ragan, who'll be playing Frank "Frankincense" Pontipee, the second youngest Pontipee brother, come to introduce himself, how very nice.

He was a handsome blonde man about six-feet tall dressed in a stylish red outfit of parachute pants. I introduced myself and thanked him for coming over, and assured him we'd be great together, which we were, but it was getting late, and we all had to find somewhere to eat so I'd see him tomorrow!

We all met up the next morning in a large rehearsal hall and we would also have the stage available for us to work on as well. Debby was pretty and very nice. Her costar was Larry Guittard, as Adam, a nice-looking gent with a very good singing voice. Others in the cast included Jani Mussetter as Liza, the two LaChance siblings, Manette as sexy Dorcas, and her younger brother, Steve, as Caleb, and his girlfriend in real life, Valerie Miller as Ruth, his love interest in the show. The twins were Jeff Reynolds and Jeff Calhoun as Ephraim and Daniel, with a number of other dancing talents as the suitors and Pontipee brother understudies.

Rehearsals began in earnest as we only had two weeks to pull the show together before opening night in Akron. We should've had three to four weeks but that is the time frame we were given, and we had to work hard and fast. Our fun and personable choreographer, Jerry Jackson, was stressed even though he had his trusty assistant, Pepper Clyde with him.

To make matters worse, about five or six of us came down with strep throat as we were constantly sweating in rehearsal with our ten-pound practice skirts, and then outside in the summer humidity that I wasn't used to at all. Our hotel room maids would turn up our air conditioning and we all came home to freezing hotel rooms, plus there was the stress of too little time.

Jerry had to squeeze the six of us into a taxicab and get us to a doctor to get us well FAST. Everything about that preparation period was fast and stressed.

We finished rehearsals and the result was kick-ass. We had a great opening and run in stinky Goodyear Tire Akron. Next, they bused us a few hours away to Columbus, home of my friend and roommate in L.A., Sha Newman. Her mom Margerie "Mother Newman" was just the best. Sha was adopted and you could not have had a better mom. Sha was so fortunate. Anyway, Terri Homberg, D. Scott Davidge, and I were all invited to spend our two-week run in Columbus at her home, and Terri and I slept in Sha's childhood single beds in her old bedroom. (Hey, I had those, one for a sleepover, remember?)

Scott slept in the spare room even though he and Terri were an item. However, the last week in Akron, Scott had become enamored of another cast member named Katherine, who was a gymnast in our show, and a bride understudy. He was no longer interested in Terri and dropped her like a hot potato. Terri was madly in love with Scott, and this was not good, especially with her and Scott under one roof. It was so uncomfortable that Marge told Scott she thought he should leave and get a hotel room.

Terri was in deep grief, and it was hard on all of us. Scott left, and things get markedly better.

We bought Marge and her friend tickets to see the show. She threw a party for the entire cast, and Larry and David were with us, so they came too. Marge Newman was a home economics major in college and a great cook, so she and her friend made all the food, and we brought the wine and beer. It was so generous of her.

There were fireflies in Columbus in the back yard at night, so Marge gave me a jar so I could catch some and watch them. I was just mesmerized as I had not grown up with them in Washinton State.

She also let us drive her car back and forth to the theater every night. All we had to do was pay for gas, which we did. I considered her like a second mom, especially with the state my own mother was in. It was hard to leave her and go to the next city, but I would see her with fair frequency, with her daughter as my roommate and friend.

Dayton was our next city and physically the cutest-looking city so far. I told Terri, no offense, but I wanted to get a room of my own. I could afford to, since we had saved money in Columbus with free lodging. The vibe was still so thick with tension between Terri and Scott that I started hanging out with Nancy Fox and Jani Mussetter, who had a great sense of humor.

We get to our final destination of Flint, Michigan, and we are all in the same hotel, a Holiday Inn about ten minutes north of Flint. It was in the countryside, as that is what was closest and affordable. It was fairly hot and humid in Flint in late July, but the Holiday Inn did have a big pool out back for us to spend our time in during the days.

We also played this silly game that was popular at the time, a board game called *Pig Mania*. There were two little plastic pigs in a dice cup that you tossed on the board and depending what position they landed in you moved so many spaces on the board to win and reach the end.

The big points position was "makin' bacon," one pig on top of another. This and swimming kept us from going crazy. We were isolated in the middle of fucking nowhere. We had Denny's attached to the Holiday Inn where we all ate, and we had a convenience store where the bus would stop for us after the shows to pick up snacks, cereal, and liquor or beer. There would be auto workers getting off their shifts from a Ford plant close to us buying lots of Mad Dog 20/20, and I was sort of sick to see that. It was such rotgut booze.

Things were really bad between Scott and Terri, and it was affecting our entire cast when we ate dinner after the show at Denny's. I think Scott felt guilty for leaving Terri, who was there constantly, just like having an office romance and still having to work with the person you broke up with day after day.

Scott started getting drunk and loud at night, and it became somewhat embarrassing for all of us, so Larry and David had a talk with him and he did stop, and I was relieved for him. I wanted him to retain his job, and go to Broadway with the show, and yes it was decided that we were going! Debby had done a lovely job, we'd gotten good reviews, and Kaslan Productions were on board to produce us. A bride on Broadway at last! Most of us were assured of continuing on, but some were not, and we were told for now to keep that discreet. After eight days in Flint, we all flew back to either L.A. or New York to be contacted about the national tour in a couple of months.

CHAPTER THIRTY

BROADWAY BOUND

It was a waiting game for a couple of months. I am busy with dance classes, go on some commercial auditions, clean our apartment, take care of kitty, Archie, and try to remain confident.

I started to run low on funds and I still had unemployment, but I needed more money to hold out for the national tour starting rehearsals about the first week in November. Sha suggests I take out a bank loan and tell them it's for car repairs. It works, and I get $1,000 to tide me over.

I got news through the grapevine that Valerie and Steve LaChance will not be going on the national tour, so now there is a need for one new bride and another Pontipee brother. Craig Peralta and I want Sha to join us, so we talk to Larry and David, and she goes and meets them. They like her, and she is chosen as Ruth, and supposedly they have come up with a very talented man from New York, Lara Teeter, as Caleb.

Larry and David decide that Terri Homberg is not a strong enough dancer to play a bride on Broadway, so they bring back Laurel Van der Linde from a previous company of *Seven for Seven.* Scott Davidge doesn't want Terri on the tour either, as he is still with his new girlfriend and it will just cause unwanted stress. They bring another female cast member on board to be Debby's understudy, Cheryl Crandall. They also hire a new full-time understudy, Gino Gaudio, for Adam. They will both be townspeople and have bit parts in the show.

There is a new Adam for reasons unknown, at least to me, and his name is David James Carroll, and or D.J. Carroll. He is a gorgeous specimen of a man and reminds me of Errol Flynn with his attitude, but more fun. He's gregarious and was a competitive swimmer and has a swimmer's body. He grew up with a silver spoon in his mouth, as his dad was the vice president of the Lipton Tea Company. David was also the costar of the play *Deathtrap* on Broadway, and in the musical *Chess* and *Oh, Brother!* before he got the costarring role of Adam in our production of *Seven for Seven*, opposite Debby. He also had supporting roles on TV, including *Knots Landing*, which Larry Kasha produced, so Larry knew him from that.

That was our Broadway company, and everybody stuck it out all the way through the nine-month national tour to our untimely end, but let's just go on the road for a while, shall we?

We did have to start rehearsing at the beginning of November for almost four weeks. At least we had plenty of time this time. My partner, Michael Ragan, and I inherited what is called the "big lift" in the Spring dance, the most difficult lift in the show out of many—but it is our job assignment, so we give it our all.

While we were rehearsing, we made a commercial for the show, and we get paid for that, as well. We rehearsed at a studio in L.A. on 3rd Street, and here is our route for the next nine months: San Diego, Seattle, Chicago, Detroit, San Francisco, Los Angles and FINALLY New York and Broadway, a true zigzag of a national tour, but all big cities and all big theaters.

We are all getting along just swell, and Debby is really remarkable as she has her first child out of what would be four in total—Jordan—who is barely a year old, and he comes to rehearsals with her husband in tow every day.

Her husband is the cute and hilarious Gabri Ferrer, son of José Ferrer and Rosemary Clooney, but he is not in the entertainment industry. He is an artist, a painter, but at this time, he's a full-time dad and househusband so Debby can work. He's a non-egotistical modern guy who wants their family to work.

Gabri is down to earth and so is Debby. One day the brides were rehearsing the opening song and dance, "Wonderful, Wonderful Day" with Debby, and I smelled some fairly pungent B.O., and I said, "I think somebody forgot their deodorant," as it was pretty strong. Then Debby says, "Oh it's me Linda, I didn't have time to wash my leotard last night because Jordan wouldn't go to sleep."

We all laughed, and she still had B.O., but we didn't have to work with her all day long, she went to rehearse with D.J., so he could enjoy her B.O. too!

Now it was time to go down to San Diego for three weeks and open the production over the Christmas holidays. I gave Archie to my friend Robert DeCapua to take care of again, and we had a subletter, Tony Cappola, at our big old apartment, as Sha and I were both gone. This is what many gypsies did with their apartments when they were on the road, and it worked very well and saved everyone money. Marge and Jack Tygett came to see Sha, Scott, and me on opening night, and they were filled with pride for us. We were filled with joy that our teachers and mentors got to see us, especially Marge, as she had been battling breast cancer on and off for a few years, but she was still standing.

Jani offered me a place to stay with her at her grandparents' townhouse, in another set of twin beds from her childhood, how nice. I was blessed again with free room. We were making $1,000 a week and had a $600 a week per diem, and what we'd all been told to do was sock the salary away and live off the per diem, so it was doable.

We also had Secret Santas and got other people in the cast Christmas gifts as well. I bought Gami and Gampi (Jani's name for her grandparents) tickets to our show and Lara Teeter bought all of the brides a pair of knee socks. I used those for YEARS.

Up to Seattle next and the 5th Avenue Theater. Many people from my hometown including my family members and friends in Bremerton came to see me. It was a fun, wild scene for me, plus the Seattle area went crazy for the guys who played the brothers. They were SOOOO handsome with their long hair, dyed red. They were chosen for their looks as well as talent for sure! We also had a restaurant hangout downstairs from us called the Goose, that came in handy after the shows for guests and our fans. We really did have a big following, mostly of young moms and their preteen to teen daughters who came to see the show several times and wrote the brothers fan letters that we posted on our bulletin board.

We had a very posh opening night party, which my sister and brother attended, and then the next day, the *Seattle Times* interviewed me, and it took up half a page of the newspaper, along with a very attractive and large photo of me—same thing with the *Bremerton Sun* newspaper in my hometown. An old boyfriend in Seattle found me and we went on a couple of dates, until I found out he'd lied to me about his marriage, telling me he was divorced.

Nancy Fox and I had brought our snow skis along with us, as we could have one other item beside our Equity trunks—yes full-size trunks, and Laurel Van der Linde had her cats! Nancy organized a rental van that we all chipped in and paid for to go skiing at Snoqualmie Pass.

First, though, I had to go see my grandmother, Freida, which was a fortuitous decision as it would be the final time I saw her. She now had such bad dementia that she didn't even recognize me and could not speak. Some in-laws were taking care of her for us, and we did pay them very well.

The skiing was great, with powder snow, and my dance partner, Mike Ragan, joined us, too. He was a skilled skier. Some just went up to enjoy the Mountain Lodge for the day. Seattle was our most enjoyable city and venue, with sold out shows and the love pouring in. I bought my mother a ticket, along with two friends from high school, Bart Bruckman, and Mark Carter, and they brought her, as she was in the throes of bi-polar mental illness and needed escorting. It was very kind of them. All too soon, a month went by, and it was time to move on to Chicago, in February, for a month. We were all sad to leave and David James was hilarious, faking crying and whining, "I Don't want to go to the EEEEEEERIE Crown," our next theater—the big barnlike Arie Crown. But we had no choice, it was our next booking.

Chicago was FREEZING with the windchill coming off Lake Michigan, but this time I had my lynx dyed fox fur, chubbie, to keep me warm. The first time was eight years ago with my rabbit fur jacket that I'd bought with the Bookends. There is almost nothing that keeps a person as warm as real fur in severely cold weather, but the cast were out buying heavy ski jackets and wool coats as fast as they could, real fur being too expensive for most. Chicago in winter is very brutal, and so was the Arie Crown Theater.

The Arie Crown sat 5,000, a BIG ASS BARN of a theater, and we could barely see the first few rows of the audience beyond our orchestra pit. It would be our largest venue on the tour. It had no intimacy about it, unlike our previous theaters. It would've been better for big rock concerts with loud bands like Skynyrd, the Stones, or Led Zeppelin, not a non-electric, old-fashioned musical. Hence, we didn't get great reviews, and at 5,000 seats, we surely never sold out. But we did start to fool around more and had some great times with each other!

Sha and her love interest and partner in the show, Lara Teeter, slowly but surely became a showmance, as Sha and Steve Canyon Kennedy parted ways. That was enjoyable to see, and they were rooming together now.

Jani Mussetter and I were becoming tight girlfriends as we had the same edgy sense of humor. One of our favorite things to do in our winter costumes was to stand and pretend to get ready to give each other a romantic kiss while holding each other in an embrace. The angle of our mouths and faces looked incredibly realistic, and all the young men in our show just loved for us to do this. It was particularly humorous, as we'd been kidnapped by the Pontipee brothers and we were all horny, waiting for the Spring thaw. That's when Milly would let all of us do a big rite of spring dance. The dance had my scary big lift, a 180-degree arabesque on Michael Ragan's shoulders, dropping me into a hold, a back attitude on one leg with a front extension on the other, twirling downstage with a front développé lift, then running off the stage in my fucking 15-pound skirt.

Jani and I also did wacky things on matinee days like put on the Pontipee brothers' lumberjack clothes and fake beards and take pictures backstage, with their fake rubber axes. Another good one was me lifting my first act 15-pound prairie woman skirt to expose my pantaloons and Jani pretending to give me head.

Our dresser would take pictures of us doing all this wacky shit, she was soooo great. I do not remember her name and she has probably gone to that dressing room in the sky by now, but she got a kick out of us and our salacious tomfoolery. She had to meet me at the side of the stage at the end of the big barn raising/hoedown dance as I was always a sweater and I was so sweaty I could not see. She helped me with a towel to wipe off my face. I would reapply almost all of my makeup during the 20-minute intermission.

About halfway through the Chicago run, one of the suitors, Jim Horvath, invited us to a party at his parents' house in a nearby suburb. We took vans out to the party, which was at a lovely, large home that had a piano that we could enjoy and sing songs.

At the start of the dinner, Nancy Fox and I were requested to bring out a roasted whole pig with an apple in its mouth on a platter, each carrying one end of the platter. There was applause for us, but I felt sorry for the piggie, of course, although I did eat some later.

We went to bowling night with the *Pirates of Penzance* cast that was also playing the other roadhouse in Chicago—many touring shows share dates in the same cities. I went mostly to support my team players as I absolutely SUCKED at bowling.

Jim Belushi was playing the Pirate King and Peter Noone of Herman's Hermits was playing the younger male lead. Jim Belushi showed up with some of the other pirates, but no Herman's Hermit. Afterwards, Jim invited us to another bar, but I was tired and begged off. I did offer him my sincerest condolences about his brother's death about five weeks or so before that and told him that his brother had come to my house for a magazine interview with my ex-boyfriend, Al Kooper. He thanked me and said he was getting through the grief as best he could. What a loss for the entertainment industry, and so young.

We tearfully said goodbye to our dear dresser, a lady who gifted Jani and me with vibrators, as we were frequently and openly talking about how horny we were.

Now we were off to another cold Eastern US city, Detroit, for SIX WEEKS, but that was because we were going to be doing two shows at once for two weeks. It was much to our surprise, until the week before we left Chicago, when the brides and brothers were called to a special meeting. It would be fun, exhausting, and more money for us!

CHAPTER THIRTY-ONE

THE DEBBY BOONE TV SPECIAL NBC 1982

Debby had done one TV special in 1980 called *The Same Old Brand New Me* for NBC, and she was under contract to do another one for the network in 1982, and they had grown impatient, or so it seemed. Geez Lord, I mean Deb was starring in a Broadway musical and was a new mom to one year old Jordan. At least she had Gabri on the road with her to help take care of Jordan.

We had a meeting with Debby, Kaslan Productions, and some NBC TV peeps who told us they'd like us to costar with Debby in a special about a troupe of gypsies doing what we were doing: a national tour of a show going to Broadway, in hopes we'd be a hit!

We would all be doing some more contemporary dance routines, more disco jazz, and some traditional musical theater routines—singing, dancing, and some spoken lines, and we'd get costar billing. The pay was $2,000 for the two weeks. We'd be rehearsing *One Step Closer* in the daytime and performing *Seven Brides* at night, along with the two matinees, also earning us $1,000 a week and $600 per diem. For me it was no brainer. The twelve of us said alrighty then, though David James Carroll and Nancy Fox respectfully declined, as it was just not their cup of tea.

I stayed at an older but elegant hotel, the St. Regis, right next to the Fisher Theater where we were playing, while most of the cast stayed at the more modern Renaissance Center Hotel farther away. I was at the point where I just needed a break from the cast. It was the right choice with this double workload situation. We always had a choice of about three hotels that gave the cast discounts, and this was a huge, big room with classic decor. Jani and DJ were also in the hotel, and we all had private rooms now.

Most of us had never been to Detroit before, and driving on the bus through the city on the way to our hotels from Chicago to Detroit, we could see the ruins of the 1967 race riots that had happened fifteen years earlier. One thousand buildings were burned to the ground, and the city was still in the process of recovering, just about everywhere.

There were also patches of snow on the ground as it was just the beginning of March, and with grey skies it gave off a spooky, ominous vibe. Jani came to my room, and we just stared out the window and made a pact not to go outside without each other for a few days. Jani said, "Rats the size of Dachshunds," and there might have been some.

We started *Seven Brides* at the Fisher the next day, and the theater was much warmer, much nicer inside than the Arie Crown and not nearly as big, thank God, and we could see the first few rows easily. The walls were very ornate like the gorgeous 5th Avenue Theater in Seattle, and it would be a pleasure working there for six weeks.

The rehearsals for *One Step Closer* were put off for another week, so we had two weeks to just do *Brides*. I turned 29 on March 13th and DJ threw me a surprise party with just selected members of the company, most of whom I WAS close to, but not some. I do apologize for that, Manette and Debby, if you ever read this, but I did appreciate the party, nonetheless. I got some G-strings, vibrators, one nice pair of underpants, and a bottle of White Shoulders cologne from DJ, as he knew it was my favorite.

Two of the gay boys pitched in and bought me the "Joy of Lesbian Sex" with illustrations on how to perform cunnilingus on your fellow Lesbian—I think in hopes that Jani and I would progress to that. We were and are definitely heterosexual, but it was an educational read.

We started rehearsals for Debby's special in the daytime in an old warehouse with a large rehearsal room on the second floor, close to the Fisher Theater, so we could deal with the two shows.

Our choreographer was the very sweet Scott Salmon, who I'd worked for on the Leif Garret TV special in '79. He was so easy to work for. The opening dance number entitled "One Step Closer" was going to be done partially on some platforms, and there was only room for Debby and eleven dancers, so someone, ME, had to bow out. Many of the other cast members had not done as much TV or movies as I had, so I volunteered, but requested more acting if possible, and it was, and I did.

We did a song with Debby that was mostly singing and pretending to go from nightspot to nightspot in Detroit's Greektown, and I was given a good couple of lines to deliver to the group during "Gotta Get Some Sleep." That was a night shoot and the only time we were all exhausted, as we stayed up until about 3am, going from location to location outdoors, and it was also fucking freezing. Gabri had left baby Jordan with the nanny, yes, they did have a road nanny, and he portrayed a drunk walking down a dark street at the end of the song. He was hilarious.

We had an early morning call at 9am, so Manette came and slept over with me, as she was all the way downtown at the Ren Center and I was very close to the rehearsal hall where we'd be shooting our big disco routine with Debby.

We went and got into costumes and make up, and the makeup lady let me lie on a cot and nap while she put my makeup on, even my mascara. I hadn't mentioned that Pete Menefee, from my *Brady Bunch Variety Hour* series was our costume designer, and what a joy for me. I just adored him, of course. He made all the exhaustion of that day better by just being there.

It was such a fun production number for all of us to dance, with sexy and very hip 80s costumes. We danced to the disco song "Dance, Dance, Dance, Dance" and it came off very well. Our costumes were terrific, in tones of bronze, oranges, and golds. It was then time for naps, before we had to go to the Fisher and do *Seven Brides* that night.

The following morning, I got an early morning call in my hotel room. It was my sister Kathy calling from Bremerton to tell me my dear grandma had departed this earth. I had gotten to see her at our in-laws in Olalla who were taking care of her, but she had such severe dementia she just walked back and forth in a robotic manner and looked straight ahead even though my sister kept telling her "Grama, Linda's here!" But she couldn't speak either. I did get to put her to bed and kiss her goodnight.

She had been so good to me, more like my mom than my mom. So, I told Kathy I'd have to speak to our road manager Dean and Larry Kasha, but my understudy was already on stage, as I shared her with Nancy Fox and Nancy had gone home for a few days to deal with some personal issues and she wouldn't be back for a while. Plus, I had about three more days work on the TV special, so I told her I'd get back to her later that day. This was going to be a stressful clusterfuck, there was just no getting around it.

There was one understudy per every two brides except for Debby, who had her own. So, what had to happen was another understudy had to go on for me that belonged to another set of brides, and that's what happened—not my understudy but Sha and Laurel's understudy learned my part over the next three days, and I called my sister and told her to put grannie on ice, I'd be there in about four days. I had to pay $2,000 for the funeral and casket as they only accepted cash or a check and nobody in my family had that to spare but me.

The last thing I had to do in Debby's special was a mini-monologue about leaving show biz and opening up a nice boutique, which preceded our last big production number sung by Craig Peralta and Debby, about him opening up a shoe store called "Is It Shoes or Is It Shows." I had more spoken lines in that—it was really clever and a good finale with a big showbiz kick line.

When asked who I'd like to say my monologue to, I asked for Pete Menefee instead of one of the brides or brothers. Why? Because Pete had been Harvey Johnson in the movie *Bye Bye Birdie* and that meant a lot to me, and he also made me less nervous.

I flew out to Seattle and got picked up by my sister and we went to the funeral home with my checkbook in hand to pay the undertaker. The next morning was the funeral, open casket, and some little old ladies singing "Bringing in the Sheaves," which was grandma's favorite hymn, and we had neighbors and friends there comforting us. We went out afterwards for margaritas and Mexican food and then I had to get back to Detroit the next morning to finish the run in Detroit. I felt like I'd aged about ten years that month, it was just so much to deal with.

Next up was San Francisco and the Orpheum Theater. Once again, out of our list of three hotels, I stayed in a small boutique hotel all by myself, because like Greta Garbo, "I vant to be alone."

One Step Closer aired on NBC on the first Monday we were there, and it was really good. We all went to Debby's hotel and had snacks and drinks and watched it together in a conference room on a large TV. It was really entertaining, and I was proud of it for all of us. Jimmy Coco and Dionne Warwick were the guest stars, and I got credit on some sites as a guest star as well. But I was just happy to get my name in the credits, and it was the best thing I ever did on TV. Thank YOU, Debby. When I got back to my little hotel, the desk people congratulated me and looked at me like I was a star, how cute!

San Francisco went pretty fast, and even though we were situated outside of the Tenderloin district, I still had to be on the lookout for homeless, drunks, and drug addicts while walking to and from the theater.

Evita was in town, playing the Golden Gate. After their sit-down engagement in L.A., they were now the first national tour. I had drinks after our shows with Scott Holmes and heard that Steve Canyon Kennedy had moved on to the star of the show, Loni Ackerman, and they were now a couple (they would eventually marry and are still married to this day), and Sha had moved on to Lara Teeter as her new showmance.

Debby had brought in a new director from New York, Grover Dale, who was married to Anita Morris and had been in the original *West Side Story* and was the actor Tony Perkins' ex-lover. Tony Perkins and Grover had both gone through electric shock therapy, and had become heterosexual, for a while at least. Tony had married Berry Berenson, sister of Marisa Berenson.

Grover was a scathingly interesting man, tall and good looking. He would help us a lot because we hadn't had a real director, just Larry Kasha, our producer. We needed a real director to succeed on Broadway.

FINALLY, we got to L.A. and home to our own apartments, my cat, and my 240Z, for a month. We were downtown at the Dorothy Chandler Pavilion, a beautiful modern theatre.

Grover started to remake the entire show and added a musical number for the Pontipee brothers in San Francisco that had been cut from the beginning of the run. It was called "Get a Wife," and it showcased the shirtless brothers in their fake beards, chopping wood with rhythmic axe-swinging. It was so damn good. And Debby had started to put more grit into her fights with Adam, and her acting was really improving because of it.

We had a good opening night and a big glamorous opening night party with the press there snapping pictures.

I was in the buffet line with Pat Boone, who told me how proud he was of Debby. Michael Kidd was there, too, and told me that he had tried to hire me as Minnie Fay for a production of *Hello, Dolly!* with Dick Van Dyke as Vandegelder. He'd left a message with my answering service when I was still with Al Kooper. It mysteriously never got to me. It made me so sad, as I would have loved doing that role and working with Michael and Dick Van Dyke, although I'm not sure the production ever happened.

Manette and I had our picture taken together and it appeared in a nice article in *The Hollywood Reporter.* During the run, I had dozens of friends from other shows come and see me and come backstage and that was very special for me. We were adding rehearsals a lot and constantly changing spoken lines on a semi-weekly basis. We did this so much that we all worried we'd fuck up and do the previous day's lines, but somehow, we never did.

Fred, the director of our *Seven Brides* commercial, was shooting a Wrangler Jeans commercial, which was called

"Dancing Girl." It was being shot in L.A., and he let us audition for it, all the brides and brothers who wanted to, doing the Texas two-step with a partner.

The audition was in the daytime so we could go. I had gone out to dinner a couple of times with Fred, and he did like me. He was a nice man, about 45 years old, and looked kind of like Victor Mature.

Not all of the brides and brothers went to the audition. They didn't have anyone dance with a partner—they just lined us up in a couple of rows with other models sent from agencies and checked us out. I was thinking, "Why didn't my commercial agent send me?"

The client chose Janet Jones, the beautiful Mrs. Wayne Gretsky and David James, as the lead dancing couple. Then they chose my very handsome Pontipee brother Michael Ragan as one of the other two men, and two other females from other agencies to dance with them. The rest of our cast was let go. The chosen would just stay at the dance studio at Moro Landis and rehearse the Texas two-step and then film it the next day.

A few hours later, I got a call from Fred, and he told me that the partner that was chosen for Michael could not dance, so she was asked to leave. Fred had told the clients that he knew I could, and he'd like me to be the replacement. So, a wardrobe gal called me, got my sizes and measurements and told me to report to some country western bar in Hollywood the next morning at 7am for hair, makeup, and costume.

I was so happy. It was a national spot and maybe it would run this time, unlike my McDonald's national commercial! My partner showed me the Texas two-step, and I grasped it in about fifteen seconds. It was so easy compared to what we did in *Seven Brides*—it was like a vacation, not a job. My Wrangler outfit included turquoise jeans and a turquoise and white checkered Western-style shirt, and I had big curls and big hair, very countrified, yee haw!

All we did was the Texas two-step forwards and backwards, with Janet and DJ center and we other two couples on either side, fairly tight together, dancing to some hokey country instrumental song on a floor covered in saw dust. This took all day long with a break for lunch, which was catered, of course. ALL commercials are catered, as are most movies, because they don't want you to leave the set, since time and lighting is tight.

We shot until almost 6pm on a weeknight and then Fred had to release us as DJ, Michael, and I had a show to do, and had to get there by 7pm. The commercial DID start running about a month later and ran sporadically all the way through 1982. The three of us made approximately $6,000 for the one-day shoot.

You see, my darlings, if you can snag a national commercial that runs, it's the best money per second an entertainer can make. That's why you want to get yourself a good commercial agent whether you are a singer, dancer, actor, or all three. Hobbies that are athletic are a plus, as stunt people aren't always used, depending on the product and storyline of the ad.

CHAPTER THIRTY-TWO

WE'RE A MISS NOT A HIT, AND LIVING IN NYC

In the middle of June we left L.A. for our big Broadway opening and hopefully a long run. Those of us from L.A. are staying at The Mayfair Hotel in the theater district, within walking distance of the Alvin, our theater on West 52nd St.

We started rehearsing the morning after arriving and opened a preview run the night after that for three full weeks. We are doing extra rehearsals constantly and still changing things, but "Get a Wife" was once again removed from the beginning of the show, and I really think if that had been our opener, we would have succeeded.

Our sets were not up to par for Broadway. We had lost a backer in Chicago, and we desperately needed sets that just glided in and out like the ones in *Dreamgirls* or *Nine*. We had a forest of trees that were made from thin cloth that moved when we ran through them in act two. We had a cabin set that had to be rolled onto the stage manually. The only exciting set piece we had was a $25,000 mechanical horse that moved its legs and was attached to our wagon in the kidnap/avalanche scene.

But we had sold out houses and the audiences seemed to like us a LOT! People I knew from other shows I was in came to see us, including Andy Gayle from Music Circus. Al Kooper and Kitty Bruce, Lenny's daughter, came but had nosebleed seats in the second balcony, as they didn't tell me they were coming until right before the show.

Al was shacking up with a groupie and was actually living in New York by coincidence, and it was nice to see them both. The next morning, Al and I met for breakfast, and he told me he had stopped going to orgies as there was this new deadly venereal disease called AIDS that was killing the sexually promiscuous, especially gay males. Anyway, I congratulated him as it would probably save his life, and that was the last time I actually saw him, although we'd speak on the phone from time to time.

About a week into the previews, I'd decided that no matter what happened I wanted to stay in New York for a few months and get the full NYC experience.

I asked around the company and Manette had a friend she did *Dancin'* with, Gayle Benedict, who was looking for someone to sublet her apartment while she was in Japan doing *Dancin'*. She was Bob Fosse's dance captain and was still working with the show. She had four cats and if I took care of them, I'd get $200 off the $800 a month rent. I liked cats. I missed mine, didn't I? And she was leaving in five days, so the timing couldn't have been more perfect.

She'd be gone until the beginning of October, so basically another three and a half months—that should work, and if I wanted longer or needed it, I'd find another sublet. She also gave me Bob Fosse's private phone number if I wanted to ring him up and go audition for him. *Dancin'* still had a Broadway company, but I just couldn't do it knowing Bob's attraction for some of his female dancers. I accepted the phone number, but I never used it.

My apartment in L.A. had Tony Cappola in it. It was a fantastic way of gypsies helping fellow gypsies. So I moved my Equity trunk up to the 12th floor of a 15-story apartment building. It was a small one-bedroom, with a tiny kitchen, a living room, and dining area, also small, but at least the ceilings were high. My bedroom had a wall-mounted TV and a queen-sized bed where I'd sleep with the four cats every night.

After three weeks of previews, we were ready, now or never, but exhausted from all the changes that finally had ended the day before. I remember lying flat on my back on the stage for notes the afternoon of opening night and falling asleep. Grover came over and poked me gently with his foot and said, "Wake up, Linda." So, we rehearsed something and then I went back to get my evening wear for the opening night party, as we were having that, of course.

My dressing room was full of telegrams and flowers but there was a vibe of doom and gloom. We were all wishing each other break-a-leg but when we went to have the opening night cast circle of love and positivity that Larry Kasha always called us to, he did not want to do it and when we did it, he was very unenthusiastic. Something negative was definitely going on.

We were ALL nervous for our opening night on Broadway despite having dragged it across the country for the past nine months. When Michael Ragan and I did the big lift with my 15-pound skirt hanging in his face, I almost blacked out and we didn't hold it in a handstand arabesque long enough, but we pulled it off only because Michael was such a good partner. We did get a standing ovation at the end, but I suppose every show on Broadway got one on opening night.

We all got dressed to the nines, and Jani, my date Brian Robert Taylor, and I rented a limo as there were two parties to go to that night. Brian had flown out from L.A. to support me and his friend Jeff Reynolds, one of the Pontipee twins in our show.

Our actual party was at an elegant private room in a restaurant with good food and drink but VERY quiet, no excitement, and almost dour. After about forty-five minutes we left for the second party at Studio 54, the real Studio 54. It was Anita Morris night, and Grover had gotten us all in.

Anita was up on the balcony with spotlights on her and disco music playing, being touted by all of us below along with all of the others that were there. Grover was down below and we all wanted to dance with him. We were in a circle saying, "Grover dance with me, dance with me," as Anita watched us from above, laughing. She knew who we were.

Grover just stood in the middle of our bride circle and danced with all of us! We were pooping out—it had been a looooong three weeks of previews and a tense opening night. When we left the club our limo driver told us the limo had broken down, so we had to walk back to where we were staying. My sublet was the corner of 70th between Columbus and Broadway, so not far, and I invited Brian to spend the night with me and the four cats, so he did, shhhhh!!!

During that period of time, Broadway did not want or like pop stars or Hollywood stars to ruin the purification of The Great White Way. It was Sondheim, Andrew Lloyd Webber, or anything Tommy Tune, as they were considered real and pure talent while the rest of us coming from the West Coast especially, were "fake" talent, smoke and mirrors, glamour and glitz.

We had a lot going against us as did *Little Johnny Jones* that went into the Alvin Theater just a couple of weeks before we did and failed after only five performances. They'd trucked their show across the country, many times right in front of ours.

Donny Osmond, we heard, was very good, very strong as the leading man. He was not only a strong singer, he could dance and tap, as well, but OH DEAR, he was a TV and singing star who had his own TV show for years with his sister, and many guest starring spots to boot, what talentless trash, right? I worked with him and danced behind him on *The Magic of ABC* TV special and was proud to do so. He was a cute and truly talented young man. But one man and one newspaper in New York thought otherwise and had the power to shut shows down.

Frank Rich was *The New York Times* lead critic and was loathed by many. He could be as nasty as nasty gets as you're about to read. He does not deserve my time or attention, but here is the main part of his review posted in *The New York Times* early the next morning.

"*Seven Brides for Seven Brothers* at the Alvin Theater. The hero is played by David James Carroll whose sturdy singing voice and colorless personality valiantly uphold the Howard Keel tradition. In the Jane Powell role, Miss Boone sings ably and smiles constantly in the remote rigidly ungiving manner of a veteran professional gladhander or beauty pageant contestant. The star's acting talents are minimal, but when her hair is up, and her forced good cheer is particularly frosty, one can picture her doing a rude impression of Nancy Reagan on *Saturday Night Live*."

I haven't read this in about forty years, and it sickened me then and it sickens me even more now as it is like Frank Rich had a personal vendetta against sweet Debby. It is unbelievably venomous and obviously misogynistic, and the part about Nancy Reagan is simply bizarre, as

Nancy Reagan was thirty years older than Debby and looked nothing like her. He also said that the chorus boy Pontipee brothers looked like clowns with their dyed red hair and gave them no compliments on their performances whatsoever. He did not mention the brides at all—we were fortunate to be left out of his seething, hateful rhetoric.

We went into work the next night and we all had written notices that we'd be closing in three days and five more performances, just like *Little Jonny Jones* had before us. It was a hard five performances. We were all depressed and mad. We met audience members wanting autographs at the stage door after every performance, and telling us how much they loved the show, which brought me to tears. I went to Debby and had her sign my program and she wrote, "Linda, we've done something we can all be proud of," and that is true to this day. We originated our roles on Broadway.

The last night of our performance, Lara Teeter and some of the other men in the show organized a picket line of the *Times* for the next day. Somehow, we got poster board and made signs and the entire company except Debby and DJ formed a picket line for about three hours over the next two days. Lara would do traditional Scottish Highland dancing in the middle of us from time to time, and we got noticed by the news, but nothing came of it.

But here's the end of the story: *Seven Brides for Seven Brothers*, the Kaslan book and score, has gone on for many years, with some variations on some of the songs, but basically the same script and it's been loved by audiences around the entire United States and England. I have seen some professional productions that have been done so well, one here in Sacramento at Music Circus, choreographed by the amazing Patti Colombo, with lifts that were even more amazing than the original, which was hard to beat. It makes my poor heart rejoice that it has prevailed over the last seventy-two years since Michael Kidd and his great cast made the movie in 1953. It's our karmic reward for those of us who loved it and worked so hard in it.

Life goes on. People told me for YEARS I should try the Big Apple and Broadway shows, that I'd work my ass off, that NYC would love me! I went and got some agents, commercial mostly, I had about six of them as that's what you did at that time.

I took class at STEPS and from Luigi Lewis who loved me and whose technique I'd grown up with as a child in Bremerton. But my favorite was Ronnie De Marco, who taught various styles in his dance class including musical theater. I also took tap class from ex-Rockette Mary Kay Brown at Carnegie Hall, whose warmup was always high Rockette style kicks at the bar right off the bat, but I enjoyed her tap a lot.

I developed some nodes on my vocal cords and was treated for six weeks by a specialist on the east side. Thankfully, my insurance paid for it.

After our show closed, Jani and I went to see *Amadeus*, starring Frank Langella as Salieri—he'd also starred in a recent movie version of *Dracula*. He was very sexy in the movie and Jani and I both had crushes on him. I was sitting on the bus, looking out the window at the lovely sunny day thinking, "I'd sure like to see Frank Langella today," and lo and behold he's walking down the street coming toward the bus on the opposite side, wearing cream-colored pants and shirt to match, looking very dapper. It really made my day, and was freaky as hell.

I took our conductor, Dick Parinello to the Russian Tea Room, as he had cooked for some of us sometimes on the road, and I promised I would treat him. We had borscht, Chicken Kiev, Russian Rice and, for dessert, blackberry Jello with real whipped cream, in that beautiful ornately decorated dining room.

About three times a week I'd meet Michael Ragan and Criag Peralta for dinner on Columbus where you could get every style of food you could think of and have a glass of wine or two for about twelve dollars, and it was good food—Italian, Chinese, Mexican, American, etc. The boys were living together now, and they took good care of me as I was alone a lot with the four cats. I'd meet Jani and Nancy, who were living on the east side, for shows sometimes, and sometimes we'd go standing room for $10 at the back of the first floor of the theater.

August rolled around and it was Sha's birthday. She had moved in with Lara in his bohemian bachelor pad, I think somewhere in the Village. We all pitched in and threw Sha an outrageous party. Some of the boys from our cast decided to put on a costume show for her. What a blast! They were dressed like cowboys and Tarzan with bare chests, some just in Speedos with sexy shirts, a very Chippendale's ambiance fer sure.

We'd gotten her a large sheet cake from an X-rated bakery with a large frosting penis on it. The very handsome John Hart was there from *A Chorus Line,* and he asked me on a date, which we went on the following weekend, to upstate New York, stunningly gorgeous country in summer. We took the train, and it was nice to see the rural part of the state.

There weren't many musical theater auditions to go on, and as I found out, the union required the major Broadway shows to have sporadic auditions whether they needed anyone or not—in other words, bogus auditions. Many of the shows at that time featured ethnic dancers.

We did go and see *Dreamgirls* from standing room and loved it. And then *Nine,* which I REALLY loved. It starred Raul Julia, Liliane Montevecchi, and the fabulous Anita Morris, Grover's wife, who sang and slithered her way through "A Call from the Vatican," the song she sang to

Guido. It was an extremely erotic and sexual performance. And the show remains one of my favorite musicals of all time.

Another fellow I was dating in college, Bruce Stevenson, got in touch with me as he knew I was in New York for a while, so he asked if he could visit and stay with me for a couple of days. He was studying art in hopes of becoming an art professor, so that is what he wanted to do, go to the big museums and drag me along. I liked art, I liked him as long as he didn't mind sleeping with the four cats. I only had one bed.

I was fortunate he came for the visit as I was not planning on museum hopping and I should have been, living in Manhattan, which was so culturally enriching. We went to the Whitney and the Guggenheim, which mostly had modern art works, and I loved its circular architecture.

We saved the best for the last—the Metropolitan. Keith and I had already been in 1980 when we saw the Picasso exhibit roadshow. This time the travelling exhibit was Rodin's "The Gates of Hell" with sculptures made of bronze castings. At the time I was mostly interested in classic artists with my favorite being surrealist Salvador Dali. I own a Dali litho, "Abraham Lincoln".

Bruce left after his brief visit, as he'd always come and gone in short intervals during my relationship with him, if one could even call it that. I had told him that I was tired of the whole show biz lifestyle at age 29.5 and was starting to desire a stable married relationship and possible children, but at least a husband, hearth, and home. He was not, and was still travelling around and enjoying being a bachelor, so that was that.

Now it was September, and Gayle Benedict got in touch with me and told me that I was going to have a roommate through October 1st when my sublet would be up and she would be back from Japan. Ravah Daley would be the roommate, who I had worked with on *The Smothers Brothers Show* seven years prior in 1975, so at least I knew her.

She was a sexy, attractive dancer and I guess she was coming to New York to look for work. She'd be getting her own place and just be staying until Gayle came back. She would be bringing her pilates machine with her from L.A. and she would put it in the living room and sleep on that with a mattress—no, she could not sleep with me or the four cats.

What people had told me would happen in New York for years did not happen at all. I had gone on at least a dozen commercial auditions and didn't even get a single callback.

All of the Broadway shows I auditioned for were NOT hiring at all. The one musical I auditioned for was at a regional theater in New Jersey. It was for the role of Minnie Fay in *Hello, Dolly!* They told me they wanted to hire me, but thought I would outshine their leads. I couldn't win for losing.

But as luck would have it, there was a union call for *42nd St.* and I heard it was legit, as they did need some replacements. That came from my conductor, Dick Parinello, who was playing auditions for producer David Merrick. It was just a few days before I was set to fly back to L.A. So, I went to the audition and got the callback. Of course, it was the day before my flight home. The Equity trunk was actually all packed up and ready to go.

I got to the Majestic Theater for the callback. I told the person in charge, I believe the show's dance captain, that I would only accept an Urchin role as that is what I remembered from seeing it in 1980, but I should have asked for any of the three supporting pals of Peggy Sawyer, as they became the Urchins for a part of the show. My bad. I would not accept just chorus after doing a principal dance role on Broadway only three months earlier. David Merrick was there watching this time, and after the initial singing and tap routine, I was released.

I could've done any of those roles had I asked and even Peggy Sawyer, as her vocal part was easy and brief. Stupid me. I was not familiar enough with the characters in the show. Later, Dick Parinello told me that David Merrick said I wasn't attractive enough for a part, just like he said that Los Angeles dancers were the least attractive group of dancers he'd ever seen, when I auditioned for the Los Angeles company he was supposedly starting, so I fell into that category again.

It was all good. Linda Hoxit from Bremerton had made it to Broadway as a principal in a Broadway show, originating my role—one for the history books. I was proud of myself for that. I had gotten a lot out of my New York experience. The only thing I never did was go to the Statue of Liberty, but otherwise I did so much. I need to add that living in Manhattan was almost like living in a small town. Grocery stores and shopkeepers got to know me and call me by name. Things like that NEVER happened in L.A.

So, I petted the kitties goodbye, hugged Ravah and wished her luck, and the saddest thing was hugging my big, fat, sweet, toothless doorman Earl and giving him his last tip—I think it was like $5 a week—as he hailed me a taxi.

CHAPTER THIRTY-THREE

MY FINAL YEAR IN HOLLYWOOD

I loved L.A. and was happy to be home, get my cat back, and drive my 280 Z. There was just a teeny problem. I now had a male roommate, Tony Cappola, who is such a nice man. Our bedrooms are far apart, and we both have our own bathrooms—it was a HUGE apartment. Sha had decided to stay in NYC and live with Lara for an extended period of time, and I was happy for her—it's just not what I had expected when we first got the apartment. I did have an open mind about it, so we shall see!

The day after I came back, I got a call from the extras casting director for *Days of our Lives,* one of the popular daytime soaps at that time. A lot of my friends had been working that soap and *General Hospital* as day players, doing background work, dancing in a disco, patrons of restaurants or bars, attractive young people—the soaps liked pretty people.

She'd had called me before, but this time she almost begged me to work the following day, even though I told her I had a slight cold, which was the truth. So, I said yes and showed up the next morning at the Burbank Studios in beautiful downtown Burbank.

We were doing a bar scene and there were about ten of us—five guys and five gals—hired as patrons of the bar, just sitting at the bar or doing crossovers in front of the bar. I had expected to have my hair and makeup done, but they did not have that for us, just a large hair salon and mirrors where we sat and did our own. Once again, I wasn't feeling great so that made me grumpy.

It ended up being a fun day with lots of tomfoolery, as we had lots of free time after we rehearsed. We didn't shoot until early afternoon.

The director gave me a bit to do with one of the principal actors—flirting, smiling, and doing a little wave to them as I sat on my bar stool. So, we shot it and the AFTRA rep was there policing, which, I heard, they frequently did. After the take they went to the director and producer and told them, "Linda should be upgraded to supporting actor" even though I had no lines.

They did not like that and even if I had nothing to do with it, they would not use me again as a day player extra, oh boo hoo. That was my day on *Days* as my friends put it, for $110, one and done. And when it aired, I didn't even watch it because as I stated in a previous chapter, I hated daytime soaps. Later, I did enjoy watching the nighttime soaps, especially *Dynasty* with the fighting bitches, Linda Evans and Joan Collins—always a good laugh!

About a week before Halloween of '82 I got a call from Kenny Ortega, who asked me if I would be available to do two commercials for Freixenet Champagne for Spain with *Charlie's Angels'* Cheryl Ladd. Kenny really did want to repay me for getting the Tubes produced, which was very nice of him, and he knew I was a well-trained professional dancer.

So yes, I was down for the gig right away and also my BFF Peter Tramm was dancing in it. Peter, his wife Marine, and I had just done a print ad a few days before for France, but Marine was not chosen for the commercial, so it was just Peter and me with some other dancers we knew, about five gals, five guys, and Cheryl Ladd.

We were rehearsing for one day in some sort of a warehouse with mirrors, and the dancers' call was before Cheryl's. We were trying out some choreography with Kenny, and Cheryl comes walking in from the warehouse doors to our left. She had some dance clothes on and her slightly greasy-looking hair was in a ponytail. She was dragging on a cigarette, and I liked her immediately, not the foo foo TV star that I expected. She was like "Hi, you guys, what's the haps?" Real casual, down to earth!

So, Kenny introduced us all, which was not the norm. Then we got right to work setting some steps and fitting her in. The guys would be working with her more than we girls, so we were released earlier than they were. Peter was going to meet me at my apartment in the morning, and we'd drive down together to the Queen Mary harbored at Long Beach, to film on the ship.

It was Halloween 1982. We were doing two full commercials for Freixenet for Spain for their Christmas marketing season which was their tradition every year with a new female star from the states. Other female stars that had done this were Raquel Welch and Liza Minnelli, either alone or with dancers.

The first one we shot was the traditional one, probably shown on the actual holidays of Christmas and New Year's Eve in Spain. We female dancers were dressed like the

Crazy Horse girls from the famous Crazy Horse cabaret in Paris. We all had blonde China Chop wigs on and skimpy costumes with mesh tights and fancy gold lamé jackets holding gold staffs and glasses of champagne. Cheryl was in a gorgeous black sequin skintight dress, speaking Spanish, and singing her song, "Fascination."

The second commercial had us in our own clothes that had been chosen by the costumer, whatever our hippest outfits were. Mine was from Fred Segal's on Melrose, my fave boutique at the time. We didn't dance a lot in this commercial. We crept out from behind large plants placed around a nightclub dance floor with patrons at tables, and I don't remember much else about it.

Cheryl was given her own small stateroom on the Queen Mary cuz she was the star. Kenny came to me and Peter and a couple of others from our cast and said that Cheryl wanted us to come down and have a couple of drinks with her. Peter and I tried to beg off. It WAS Halloween, even though no trick or treaters ever came to my apartment, but Kenny was really into shmoozing with the celebs over the years, part of his success and charm, so we went.

Cheryl was smoking, so at least I got to smoke, too, as I was still doing that. It was pleasant, and I could say I hung out with a Charlie's Angel and a world-famous choreographer, as that is what Kenny became from his jump start with the Tubes, through Al and me.

We stayed for about an hour and then drove home in my Z car. It'd be the last time I actually got to work with my dear Peter, who was like my younger brother and who I loved dearly. We made about $1,000, as it was a buyout. That was for both commercials, as the buyout price at that time was only $500. You can see an old copy of the commercial on YouTube if you look under "Freixeinet commercial Cheryl Ladd 1982."

November 1982, and here comes Thanksgiving, my least favorite and even bad luck holiday over the years. This one would be no exception. Growing up, my grandparents would have some of my grandmother's five sisters over, as we had the nicest house and dining room and a separate kitchen

My grandma and her sisters lived in different cities about forty-five minutes away from each other. Although not that far from each other, they were busy with their own lives, kids, and grandkids. They usually hadn't seen each other in a while, so somebody would say something to the other sister, which led to harsh words and crying, always in the kitchen. My sister and I were the only little kids there, all the rest were grownups—not so fun for us.

I had dated a man in NYC almost at the end of my time there, named Johnny Yune. He was a famous Korean comic and an opera singer, yes, an opera singer. He was a frequent guest on *The Tonight Show* with Johnny Carson because he would do his stand-up comedy routine and then sing opera with a trained, powerful tenor voice. It was hard to believe that this handsome Asian man was singing Italian opera!

Another girlfriend had befriended him in Hawaii, and he was coming to NYC to do a private performance for a group of wealthy businessmen. He invited me to come and see him as his special guest. I'd had had like one date that went nowhere the entire time I'd been in NYC, so hell yes, and it would involve food after the concert, too.

I had a table by myself with a glass of champagne and enjoyed his marvelous performance. I had seen him once on the Carson show but seeing him in person was truly amazing. I was smitten.

Afterwards, we went back to his hotel suite, I don't remember where, but it was gorgeous and had room service, extremely good Chinese food, and some Dom Perignon bubbly. And yes, I broke my own personal rule about first dates and spent the night and it was lovely, truly. Before I left the next morning, he said he'd get in touch with me in L.A. as he knew I was going back, and I gave him my information. He had a condo in the Santa Monica area near a golf course, as he liked golf. He said he'd be in touch as he was travelling for a while.

About the second week of November, he called me and invited me to a screening of a movie he starred in and produced. At the time it was called *A Fistful of Chopsticks.* It was a very funny slapstick sort of movie about him constantly getting mistaken for Bruce Lee and getting in all sorts of predicaments because of it.

We went to his condo and hung out for a while after the screening, and he asked me if I wanted to go to his sister's house and join him for Thanksgiving dinner. I said sure as I hadn't made any plans at all yet, and that was also always a conundrum when it came to Turkey Day: who's going where, who's bringing what, who's making the bird when you didn't have accessible family and also it being the WORST holiday to fly—and still is. He said he would call me and tell me what time and pick me up the.

So, I'm floating along on a happy little cloud as I thought there were no worries about the holiday.

But the days go by and no phone calls from Mr. Yune—zip, zero, nothing. The day before Thanksgiving arrives and I suppose I should've called him and said, "What up?" but I felt awkward doing that. I also consulted a couple of friends, and they said, "Aw, fuck him, come over to our celebration," but ya know, I just couldn't.

I had the wherewithal to go to Gelson's market, buy myself a turkey leg and some sides, and I just spent Turkey Day with Archie. Tony wasn't even in the apartment—he was going to a girlfriend's house for dinner. I called home and talked to what family I had, then called a couple of friends. And that was my once again bad luck holiday.

Johnny's movie came out. They'd changed the title to *They Call Me Bruce* and it was a big hit. I was genuinely happy for him and the film—it was clever and deserving of that. But I never heard from him again, and when I told some person who knew his background they said, "Johnny's been with a Korean movie star for years, and he goes back to see her a lot."

I did see him on the Carson show a couple more times and by the time Johnny Carson retired he had been a guest on *The Tonight Show* thirty-four times.

Then it was Christmas and New Year's 1982. I went home, and it was just sort of a fog for me. My grandma had died the previous February, and the house was out of control. My mom's bipolar illness had gotten worse, and my sister was doing the best she could trying to help her and our brother, who had other issues.

My sister was the executrix of the estate, and I was having an issue with her giving me a copy of my grandmother's will and that was unpleasant, and I went back to California without a copy of said will.

Welp, 1983 now and I had some hopes of maybe finding a decent relationship, but where? An acquaintance of mine set me up on a blind date with a psychiatrist friend of hers, and it was a complete disaster. He basically called me a whore when he came to pick me up for lunch and it was the worst date of my adulthood. He tried to say he was just joking, but I didn't find it funny at all.

I couldn't find any auditions that really suited where I was with my career. I auditioned for some dance jobs, but my heart wasn't in it. My Wrangler Jeans commercial was running, and I still had unemployment, so monetarily I was doing fine. I also had $40,000 in the bank from *7 Brides.*

I was taking Joe Bennett's dance class with Jani at Debbie Reynolds' studio in North Hollywood, and Jeff Goldblum was in class with us. He always danced next to me in my group, and it was a very hard technical class. Jeff was a fine actor, but it was brave of him to even take the class. We would give each other looks of exasperation a lot, and he was an unspoken buddy of mine.

Sha wasn't coming back to L.A. any time soon and although Tony was nice enough, I just felt like I didn't want a male roommate. He was cute, and popular and was dating quite a bit, and his gals coming and going just didn't jive with me.

One time, two of his dates almost ran into each other, and it was just too much drama. Ironically, the one-bedroom apartment next to ours became available, so I told Sha and Tony I just wanted to be alone for a while, but I'd be right next door. So that's what I did. It was an easy move, and friends didn't balk too much about helping me. I didn't have that much furniture, and it was only about 150-feet away.

My Bay City Roller finally came into town and came to see me in my new digs. He'd been hiding out from Clive Davis since he quit the band but finally felt safe enough to visit, almost four years later.

I made us lunch, and he gave me his solo album from England, *All Washed Up*, as it had the song he'd written for me, "Long Distance Love." It was flattering, but the song was mostly melodramatic and redundant. We had a good old-fashioned Scottish shag on my living room rug, for old times' sake, and then he left, never to be seen again by me. A short time later he married his Japanese girlfriend Peko, and they lived a sort of up and down life. I was glad it wasn't me.

My 30th birthday came as usual on March 13th, and my dear L.A. tribe threw me a party at a sushi restaurant on Sunset in a private upstairs room. Attending were The Tillet sisters, Bridget Holloman, Rrrrrroberto Decapua, Ricky Brown, Jaclyn Lombard, my professional belly dancer friend, and me. It was fun. I had asked for towels as gifts as I didn't have enough, so I got a lot of red towels, the base color of my bathroom at the time. Cindy Tillet ordered lots of saki, and it was fortunate we all made it home safely.

Over a year later, my sister finally paid me back the $2,000 that I had gladly shelled out for Freida's funeral from the probate of my grandmother's assets. But the family had a stock portfolio that would be part of our inheritance. I had requested a copy of the will at least a half-dozen times, and the most recent time she said, "Oh Linda, mom just gets everything." I knew that was not the truth at all.

My grandma had signed a codicil to the will that specifically said that if mom was diagnosed as disabled by the state of Washington, she could only have a trust fund of several thousand dollars that could only be distributed by the executrix, my sister, on the basis of need, as my mom would run through it like water the way she had always done with money for years.

So, it was time to speak to my attorney, Walter Hurst, about how to proceed. I told him what was being said to me and he asked if I knew if I were a beneficiary. I said most certainly, and my grandmother had also promised me her diamond dinner ring.

He said that the executor or executrix had a fiduciary responsibility to distribute all properties of said will and/or monies that was owed the beneficiaries or they could be sued for breach of duty.

We both felt that my sister didn't fully understand her fiduciary duty as it was her first time being an executrix. Also, all the beneficiaries should be automatically given a copy of the will. He phoned her up the very next day and explained to her that she was breaking the law and to please send me a full copy of the will by the beginning of the following week or a breach of duty lawsuit would progress. My goodness, I adored my Walter.

Welp, that sure did it. Kathy did not understand, we gave her the benefit of the doubt, so it wasn't entirely her fault. I got the will that week. What it held was quite logical. My mother would only be allotted $20K in trust for her needed expenses. She'd been a state employee for years and was covered on disability and Medicaid.

Our house should be sold and distributed three ways—to myself, my sister and my brother. Kathy had told me she could live in it rent free until she completed her Masters in math from the University of Washington and that I was not allowed in the house. But there was no mention of that in the will. Kathy was allowed to run my grandfather's stock portfolio but if one of the beneficiaries should need money from it for a good reason, i.e. health insurance, down payment on a house, or, for me, later, money for a wedding, that should be discussed by the three beneficiaries and ok'd as a sibling trio. My grandparents' household goods and furniture should be distributed four ways, although my mom was in a group home and could not use any of it.

So, eventually Kathy would do her duty, and I got what I was supposed to get, as did my brother. My grandmother's diamond ring was the only thing I never received—it had mysteriously vanished.

I was already considering moving back to Washington State, as I was really burning out on my Hollywood career, and the men I was meeting, if any at all. I thought I would have a better chance of finding a decent more family-type man and falling deeply in love instead of the fairly shallow types I was meeting, or ones where the chemistry was just not there.

My Wrangler Jeans commercial continued to run at least a couple of times a week, and I still had unemployment coming in, so I was still not desperate for money.

In April, my girlfriend Bridget called me up and said she had an audition for me that she couldn't go to, so she thought I could get it. Over the years we all did that for each other, got each other jobs if we couldn't do them. It was a commercial for a product from Japan called MamyPoco Diapers and they were looking for five mommies to dance with babies, real ones, in strollers, along with one dancing pregnant mommy, a goofy, funny dance. I don't know where she even came across the audition, but WTF? My agent sure didn't send me.

I go to the audition and there are about four Japanese gentlemen there, one of which was the choreographer/ director. They introduced themselves to me and bowed and I bowed back. The chorographer gave me some dance moves that were sort of Egyptian with the hands and told me to do them and act kind of "goofy" and facially animated. I was good at goofy and not afraid of being foolish, and they hired me right there, almost as good as my Mr. Blackwell commercial audition.

I was going to be the dancing pregnant mommy with four other mommies with four strollers with real babies dancing behind me and pushing the strollers down a sidewalk. I was the STAR!

I got measured for a maternity-style dress, and then I was told to report the following day to a residential neighborhood for the outdoor shoot. I went home and called my girlfriend Bridget and told her not only did I book the commercial, but I also got to be the star mommy, and I was going to pay her ten percent when I got paid, cuz that is what an agent would get.

The next day I go to the neighborhood of Los Feliz, a lovely, elegant neighborhood with elegant homes but a different feel than Beverly Hills. We are shooting on a sidewalk with an elegant house behind us and a lovely tree canopy above us. There is a large trailer there for me and the other four mommies with their own babies. The four strollers were parked on the sidewalk. Clever these Japanese to hire women who could do simple dancing who had their own babies for the shoot.

The stylist first puts me in a 9-month pregnancy "bump" made of foam rubber with a strap that went between my legs and fastened in the back. It was ridiculously huge, so she switched me to the 6-month "bump", and it was perfect under my red maternity dress with a white blouse.

The director/choreographer at first wanted me to come dancing down the yard of the house behind us, down a little hill with grass and hit my mark on the sidewalk in front of the babies and mommies who would leave the strollers behind and follow me in the silly mommy dance.

The problem with that was I couldn't see the ground in front of me from the baby bump on my stomach, and it was scary—I felt like I would fall. So we moved it to a section of the yard that was almost flat and that worked. When I hit my mark I would turn to my right on the sidewalk and do the goofy mommy dance forward and the mommies would dance down the sidewalk with me for a few steps, then we'd dance back and forth on the sidewalk side to side doing another goofy dance.

We rehearsed this a couple of times and then did a take, but the babies started to cry when the mommies left them! We couldn't have that. The babies were tired and needed a nap so we shut down production for ninety minutes so the babies could have a bottle and their naps, and we could all have a catered lunch.

After lunch we did more takes and that was that. They told us that the commercial would cut to product at the end with a voiceover in Japanese. You don't usually get to see the finished product like I eventually did with the Freixenet Champagne commercial.

I did end up teaching a lot of commercial TV acting classes in Seattle (hint hint) and about fifteen years later I was teaching a class with a young woman from China in it who had also lived in Japan in the 80s. I was telling my adult class about what buyouts were and mentioned the MamyPoco commercial as an example, and this gal piped up and said, "Linda, I saw your commercial, I remember you! You were so funny and so pretty in it, and it ran all the time!"

That made me emotional, as it's kind of like having a baby and giving it up for adoption when you are the principal or star and never get to see it,

I read in the trades that San Bernadino Civic Light Opera was doing a production of *Seven Brides for Seven Brothers*, and Jack Bunch was the director, who I did twelve musicals with in 1973 and 1974 at Sacramento Music Circus.

San Bernadino is a medium-sized city close to the San Bernadino Mountain range. The San Bernadino Civic Light Opera was well-known and highly thought of, but it did take about an hour and fifteen minutes each way to drive there from where I lived in the San Fernando Valley.

But I decided I want to do Sarah one final time, as I was aging out of the role for sure. And of course I could use the money, $1,000 a week for rehearsals and the run of a month. I also talked my now BFF Jani into doing it again with me, so we could carpool together, too.

Our star was Stella Parton, younger sister of Dolly by three years, and my partner was the handsome and excellent Blane Savage who had partnered many female stars over the years, on TV mostly, and been in Juliet Prowse's stage act, too. But was most known for partnering my role model Ann-Margret on stage and screen. I was lucky to have him, and I knew him from dancer parties and auditions.

So, the first morning of rehearsals rolled around, and we were working with Jack and Pepper Clyde who I had now done four companies of *Seven Brides* with as either a bride or an assistant choreographer. Now she was the full-fledged choreographer recreating Jerry Jackson's choreography, and that was all good.

About an hour after we began, Stella comes walking into the rehearsal area, and she is cute, has a voice and face like Dolly's, blonde hair but unlike Dolly, literally NO BOOBS! And she says to us, pointing at her chest, "Hi y'all, and go ahead and stare because no I don't have boobs like my sister, pleased to meet ya." Such a good icebreaker!

Things were moving along swimmingly at rehearsals. Blane was such a good partner. We still had to do the big lift in the Spring dance, and in the chase scene in act two I'd still do my Bugs Bunny jump in the air and yell "Frank" in a baritone voice, which still got the best laugh in the show.

I had my Jani with me and we were managing to do lots of salacious hijinks in our dressing room, which had now progressed to Brides in bondage and topless pictures of us in our pantaloons and bonnets, and no I won't include the pictures in this book.

Stella sounded just like Dolly and even added a couple of trills like Dolly did from time to time, and it was charming. The rest of the cast is also nice and fun and of course Jack Bunch is always so upbeat and never demanding or sarcastic as a director.

BUT ... it gets to be about the middle of the second and final week of rehearsal and dear, sweet Stella isn't off book yet. We brides especially are starting to get nervous about this as the rest of the cast is off book, polished, and ready to hit the boards.

Two nights before we open, we brides take Jack Bunch out drinking to discuss our feelings about Stella. We had already chosen one of us who could replace her, if need be. I cannot remember her name, but she had the closest vocal range to Stella, coloratura soprano, and could hit all of Milly's notes. Jack said he'd discussed it with Stella, and he had faith she'd pull through and not to worry.

Two days later, it's full dress and orchestra and sure enough, Stella knew every word of every song and spoken line and what a huge relief that was. We had a terrific opening night and a good run, with sold out houses and friends coming down from L.A. to see us.

After a month and the wearying two-and-a-half-hour commute both ways, my Sarah, who got the best review of all of the Brides on Broadway in *New York Magazine*, took her final bow at 30 years old.

In June of '83, a dear friend of mine, Dr. Alan Creed, who had stayed in my little studio apartment when I was in Aspen to help him through chiropractic school asked me to come to join him for his 40th birthday on Maui. He'd fly me to Oahu first, though, as he had some business to do there, and I could also see a couple of friends for a night, as well.

We were going to attend the magnificent, spiritual Merrie Monarch Festival, which, at that time, was held at the University of Hawaii on Oahu. It was the competition of all of the Halaus from the Hawaiian Islands in 1983.

What a treat and lifelong memory that was for me, and the All Men's Halaus where they did stronger, warrior-like choreography. It just blew my mind, as I had never seen anything like it! I encourage anybody who loves Hawaiian culture and spirituality to try and partake of the festival on Hilo where it's now done. It will enlarge your heart tenfold.

The good doctor lived in Lahaina in a remote area with nothing but the beach across the street—no restaurants or shops within walking distance. My dear Dr. Creed went to work all day long and left me alone for eight hours a day. The first day I had no food in the fridge except carrots and coconuts. He came home and took me to dinner, and I brought home a doggie bag to survive on the next day.

This happened for the next two days, and I got my last bad sunburn as I had nothing else to do but go to the beach. I stayed in the condo the last day, but I developed what is referred to as Island Fever and I practically ran to the plane to fly me back to L.A.

I just needed to get back to a continent, and I've had no desire to go back to any beach and swim ever since, even though I had a nice vacation seeing Dr. Creed. Now I only go to Santa Cruz in California and walk around the beach on the cliffs and enjoy looking at the ocean.

Back in L.A. and I am thinking about the rest of my life. I am not motivated to look for work much as I no longer want to stay in L.A. I am talking with a small group of friends who are renting a triplex and have an extra bedroom in the Seattle suburb of Magnolia. I could stay with them until I found my own place. I am seriously considering it.

Now it's August and I have many girlfriends who are August babies, so many that we have this Leo party every August for the Leo dancers turning another year en masse. Sort of like Christmas in July, but we only gave gifts to our closest friends and ALWAYS went to our favorite Mexican restaurant El Cholo on 3rd Street in L.A.

We had lots of margaritas, and we'd get so loud they'd have to ask us to please be quiet or leave, but ya know, those margaritas!

Then some of us would go ice skating, my BFF Bridget's idea as it was so hot in August. She had grown up in Alburquerque, and that was one of their summertime activities when the weather was miserably hot.

So, we did that and then went to my apartment so I could present her with her gift: a black and white kitten in a grocery bag that I found in the classifieds. She loved it and named it Oreo, and she had her for many years.

But here comes fall and inclement weather so it was either MOVE or get stuck in L.A. until spring of '84. So, I made a solid decision to move and discussed it with my friends. I went to both of my remaining agents and picked up the rest of my headshots, Zed cards, thanked them, and tearfully told them goodbye. Joan Mangum told me that if I ever came back, I could come back to her agency, which was lovely. The general rule was if you left an agency, that was it, you did not come crawling back. I am still friends with my wonderful Joan to this day.

The last few days of September, I flew a couple of the guys down who were living in the Seattle triplex, and they brought sleeping bags to sleep on my living room rug. I had reserved a small U-Haul truck and the proper chains to tow the 280Z behind it. I did not have much furniture, only enough for one bedroom and a small couch and my poor kitty Archie who would have to make another move in a cat box for two days. I got a wardrobe box for my clothes, and the rest of my household goods went into my Equity trunk and a couple of suitcases.

My friends came over to hug and kiss me goodbye and helped us pack the U-Haul and it was so fucking sad.

My landlords came over early the last morning to inspect my cleaning job and give me my apartment deposit, and away we went, with the 280Z on a tow dolly behind the U-Haul. We drove about ten hours to Redding, with a couple of pit stops to pee and eat lunch.

Then I got us a big, inexpensive hotel room with two queen-size beds and a pullout couch, where we could spend the night.

It was dinner time, and we asked the hotel clerk where we could get a decent meal, and he pointed us toward a large barn-like building a couple of blocks away. He said it was a Basque restaurant that served big group meals that was especially popular with truckers and working-class folk, as the meals were very generous and hearty.

We walked up and there were two large entry doors that were open as it was a hot day. Inside were rows of picnic-style tables and folding chairs. The tables were covered with white butcher paper. We were the first people there at about 6pm and the hostess/wait person seated us and asked us if we'd like the family-style meal for three, which came with a bottomless carafe of Rosé wine.

What a treat! A big bowl of bean and vegetable soup, lamb shanks and pork ribs for the entrée, green beans, red new potatoes and big hunks of fresh baked French bread. Of course, I was treating my movers and paying for all transportation expenses. We waddled back to the hotel room and passed out we were so tired from the day.

We got up very early, showered, had breakfast, and hit the road to Seattle with just pit stops in beautiful, very green Oregon, and then on to Seattle, to the suburb of Magnolia.

We arrived safe and sound at the triplex and then went to Dick's Drive-In and got us a bag of Dick's burgers and notoriously greasy fries to celebrate our safe trip home.

The triplex unit wasn't that big, but I just knew it wouldn't last more than a month. One of the guys who came down to help me move had a crush on me, and there was no way I wanted that. There was a certain amount of substance abuse going on at the triplex, especially with the men, and it led to bad tempers, nasty comments, and a totally unpleasant living situation.

One of the other gals and I moved out and got ourselves a really cute half-a-house situation in an old Victorian home on Queen Anne Hill, one of the seven Seattle hills. This single-family house had been made into two homes—each with two-bedrooms and one bathroom, kitchen, living and dining room, and front and back yard. Best of all ... Archie was welcome!

My dance studio in Bremerton, still run by Margie Speck, wanted to hire me but not until after the first of the year. So, I got a part time job teaching Jane Fonda-style aerobics at a health club close to us in north Seattle a few days a week for the last three months of the year.

I met a cute guy named Pat Turner there who I dated for a few months, but ironically, he was studying acting and doing local plays and wanted to move to L.A. to pursue a film career, and I wanted just the opposite for myself. So he went down to L.A., and he did work on some soaps. He looked like a blonde John Ritter, and at least he did get some work.

I basically spent the last three months of 1983 reacclimating to Washington State and the greater Seattle area, hanging out with roommate Marla, and just sort of feeling like an average human being again. I got an agent, Lola Hollowell, who was everybody's agent in Seattle at the time.

I booked two print jobs with her, one for a wind surfboard company and another for Alaska Airlines. She then sent me on an audition for a movie being shot in the greater Seattle area, the story of serial killer Ted Bundy, who I had heard of, but really knew next to nothing about.

So, I went to the audition, got some sides, and sat in the waiting room to prepare. The role is of a young woman in a bar who Ted tries to pick up, and the young woman basically tells Ted to fuck off. She does not leave with him, so she survives. Not a lot of lines but very "me," nice and strong.

I am called into the audition room and give the producers and director my headshot and resumé, and they are totally impressed and tell me so, especially because I had worked with Barry Williams, "Greg Brady" of *The*

Brady Bunch, on *The Brady Bunch Variety Show* and he would be starring as Ted Bundy in their movie!

I read the sides for them, and I get hired on the spot. I admitted to them that I really didn't know much about Ted Bundy, and they gave me the entire script to read so I would understand what a scary, murdering monster he was. I just have to return the script to Lola Hollowell's office by the end of the week, and they will pick it up.

I returned home to our half-house and told Marla about my part and the story. I also told her that I knew nothing of Ted Bundy—I'd only heard his name mentioned in the news. Marla said, "Terrible Ted and his Volkswagen murders? Everybody in Washington State knows who he is or was. He's on death row now in Florida."

Apparently, he did most of his killings in Washington State and grew up in Tacoma between Bremerton and Seattle, starting his killing spree in the U District in the Spring of 1974. He drove all over to different university areas in his VW Bug, luring young college women by pretending to have a broken arm in a sling, using crutches, and abducting them to remote areas where he would rape and brutally murder them.

The script was very graphic and violent, and I wondered why sweet, funny Barry Williams was chosen to do this very creepy, unsavory role? I got myself to a library as soon as I could and looked for images and more information on Ted Bundy and found a lot. Barry and Ted were doppelgangers, they could have been twins in some photos, so it was a typecasting choice fer sure. Anyway, the movie would be quite graphic and extremely violent, and there were only two of us in the movie that got away from Ted, all the rest were violently murdered.

I took the script back to Lola who was as pleased as I was that I got a nice supporting role. But she had just talked to the producers, and they told her that the movie still needed backers as there wasn't enough money yet, and to please be patient, filming would begin in about a month or two. This was not unusual, but it was just hard to hang in there as there was no holding fee for the chosen actors like there sometimes was.

About once a month for the next three months I'd ask Lola what was up with the Ted Bundy movie, but there was no word yet. At the beginning of '84, she was told that it wouldn't be happening as the script was just too violent. Actually, I was not surprised—just reading it made my heart race and sent shivers up my spine. I felt so fortunate to have moved to California and had my college education there at the times of his killing spree.

In 1986, there was a made for TV movie about Ted Bundy called *The Deliberate Stranger*, starring Mark Harmon. The movie was well done and not that graphic, as it was on national TV. Mark Harmon knocked it out of the park, although he didn't look that much like terrible Ted.

The funny thing is, I saw Barry a few years ago at the Stockton, California Asparagus Festival, where he was a guest celebrity, doing a meet-and-greet, and signing autographs. I wanted him to sign my *Brady Bunch Variety Hour* book that we were both featured in. The author of the book, Ted Nichelson, put me in touch with Tina Mahina, Barry's wife, and she told Barry to expect me so I could get a few private moments and a book signature from him.

When we met him, he barely remembered me, but he was very nice to me. Florence Henderson had just passed a couple of years before, and we spoke of her for a moment and how much we liked her.

I told him that I was cast with him as a non-victim in his Ted Bundy movie that never happened, and how freaky that was for me, but that I'd looked forward to seeing him in '83. He shook his head and just said, "It wasn't meant to be," and I said, "I have to agree with you, it was just too graphic, too bloody, but what a coincidence for us." Then he had to return to his fans and his autographs, and we went to see a Lynyrd Skynyrd cover band called Skynnyn Lynyrd who I became friends with. I loved how accurate they were at covering one of my favorite bands.

I know I'm skipping around, but don't be confused, dear reader, we're still in 1983, and here come the holidays. Halloween has always been my favorite holiday, but we didn't do anything and didn't have very many trick or treaters.

Then came Thanksgiving, my ubiquitous bad luck holiday, but I went with my steady Pat to his cousin's house for a big friendly fun feed, as my sister said she wouldn't be doing anything at our house, but that she'd have me over for Christmas Day, and that was fine.

Marla was managing one of her dad's chain restaurants, Captain K's, across the water in Poulsbo. She needed a getaway before Christmas, so we decided to go skiing and get a resort room at Crystal Mountain for three days and come back early Christmas Eve so we could just slide into Christmas.

It was GREAT! We had a bunk bedroom in a ski lodge at Crystal Mountain, all knotty pine that came with a free lodge cat that slept with me in our room. The snow was dry and fine, and the restaurant's hearty, hot cuisine was good. We left the stress of the holidays far behind us until we came home.

When we got home, there was an urgent message from Kathy on our answering machine, asking me to call her. I did and she answered in a very humorless tone, very serious.

She was cancelling Christmas—she just didn't feel like having it. Mom was in a group home, as her mental illness had progressed. Our brother Stan had moved to Longview, and probably wouldn't show up due to his immature party habits. If it were just me, she'd be forced to discuss the contents of the will as I was the only other family member who even had a copy, and who cared about its contents. So Merry Christmas and goodbye.

So now what? I was so shocked and hurt I could hardly think straight. I could've gone and picked up my mom and brought her over and made some food or gone out, but I was really depressed. It felt like I had gone from the frying pan of Hollywood into the fire. I knew my family was dysfunctional, but somehow, I just thought we'd all pull together and become a normal family.

Marla to the rescue. "You can come over and spend it with us at my folks' house, they won't mind, but my grandpa will be there, and he is dying, just so you know." I appreciated the offer and that I wouldn't spend Christmas alone. I had no gifts for them, of course, but we'd stop and get a bottle on the way and ride the ferry, which was always soothing and nice.

I went, and had a peaceful, relaxing holiday. I always adored Marla's mom Diane, such a sweet chill woman. Marla would soon be filing for divorce from her husband Dan, one of the triplex dwellers, and she started to discuss that with her family. They were all on board with her. Her grandpa just laid on the couch and rested and it was lovely to see Marla interact with him, this final Christmas before he passed.

Then we took the last ferry home, and it was like Christmas never happened. It had been a relief that there was no fighting in their house over the holidays, unlike mine.

The week between Christmas and New Year's, a time to reflect and collect thoughts of the coming year and just relax and chill out! And this is where my main story ends, my friends, as that chapter of my life, filled with all the craziness, success, ups, downs, tears, joy, and laughter, is coming to a close.

I went to Pat's Bar on lower Queen Anne for New Year's Rockin' Eve. I drank, kissed strangers and Pat and Marla at midnight, and had high hopes for ringing in 1984 in Seattle.

I do hope you at least found my wild ride entertaining, cuz it's a wrap. Please read "Life Aprés Hollywood" to find out the ever after, and thanks for coming along with me on this time machine to the past and my life.

LIFE APRÉS HOLLYWOOD

I make no apologies for the wild in my life—I am the WILD, a survivor who's still here and happy.

There is that saying, "You can't go home again," and I'd say that is fifty-percent true. I had forgotten that MOST men born and raised in Washington State did not like me, and many of the females were jealous. I thought that after twelve years of being gone, things would be different, but nope, not so much.

I had a dysfunctional family, one of the many reasons I left the state in addition to pursuing my career. I was always blessed to find good friends, especially in California, who still come and visit me, and I, them. You don't choose your family; you choose your friends.

I had hoped for better with my family when I moved back, but nothing in life is perfect. I got the inheritance that my grandmother's will provided, which helped me tremendously to get married and buy a house (with many pets). By the time I did find a husband and got married, I was 37 years old, and my husband was 41. I decided not to have children, as I was too old.

Some years later, at 54, my husband would have a stroke and be disabled, and I had to take care of him and work full time for the next eight and a half years.

I taught dancing at various schools in the greater Seattle area. Teaching dance properly required a lot of prep work, with fresh choreography, and it was very time-consuming hard work, but the end results were very rewarding. The "dance mom" situation was rough, and thankfully I didn't grow up with that. It ruined some student careers that could have been successful, but c'est la vie.

I began teaching acting, which was a thousand times more enjoyable. I taught mostly TV commercial acting, as I had up to date techniques that my BFF Bridget taught me, as she was making most of her income from commercials in the 90s and 2000s. It even helped me book an industrial film for Microsoft in 1999 called *Fusion,* featuring an aging hippie deadhead chasing a Microsoft CEO around like a rockstar.

I also taught scene study for film and television, and monologues that won awards in acting competitions. My students booked TV shows, films, commercials, and one, Kenny Ridwan, still has a recurring role in the TV series *The Goldbergs,* as David Kim.

My first husband, Richard, was sexy, funny, and loyal, not great with money, but we did buy a nice home, and then a condo after he had his stroke. He didn't have good health habits, but did not do cocaine or drink at all, and we were together twenty-five years until his passing.

My second husband, Alan, found me soon after Richard. We had worked at Sacramento Music Circus at the same time in 1974, but I was with Al Kooper at the time, and he was still a senior in high school. After all these years and still remembering me, out of curiosity he decided to look me up online. He found me in Seattle, through my work at John Robert Powers, as I didn't have a computer or Facebook account yet. Alan was back in Sacramento, having worked over thirty-five years in Theater Operations and Stage Management.

We began talking by phone, which eventually led to him visiting me in Seattle. We became close, and soon, he asked me to marry him. He is four years younger than me, with good health habits, doesn't smoke or do drugs, and is loyal to a fault. He's provided me with a lovely home. His career and travels had put off marriage until a later age with me, but he has done a swell job adjusting to married life. Once again, it was too late to have kids, so our dog and cats filled the void.

We've traveled extensively, going to Iceland, Scotland, England, France, Italy, Egypt, Florida, and throughout the Western United States. I don't have to work now and am retired, with SSI and a nice AEA union pension. I also do volunteer work for my other union, SAG/AFTRA. I'm back in my beloved California, Sacramento to be exact, which is truly my positive Feng Shui. People LIKE me here.

Well, that's it in a happy nutshell. I always consider all of the other countries, ethnicities, talents and mental abilities I could've been born into, but was so fortunate for this mind, body, and life. I only hope that when and if I do come back, the next life will be half as great as this one.

My best to y'all, always. Peace, love, and have a sunshine day.

Linda Caroline Hoxit

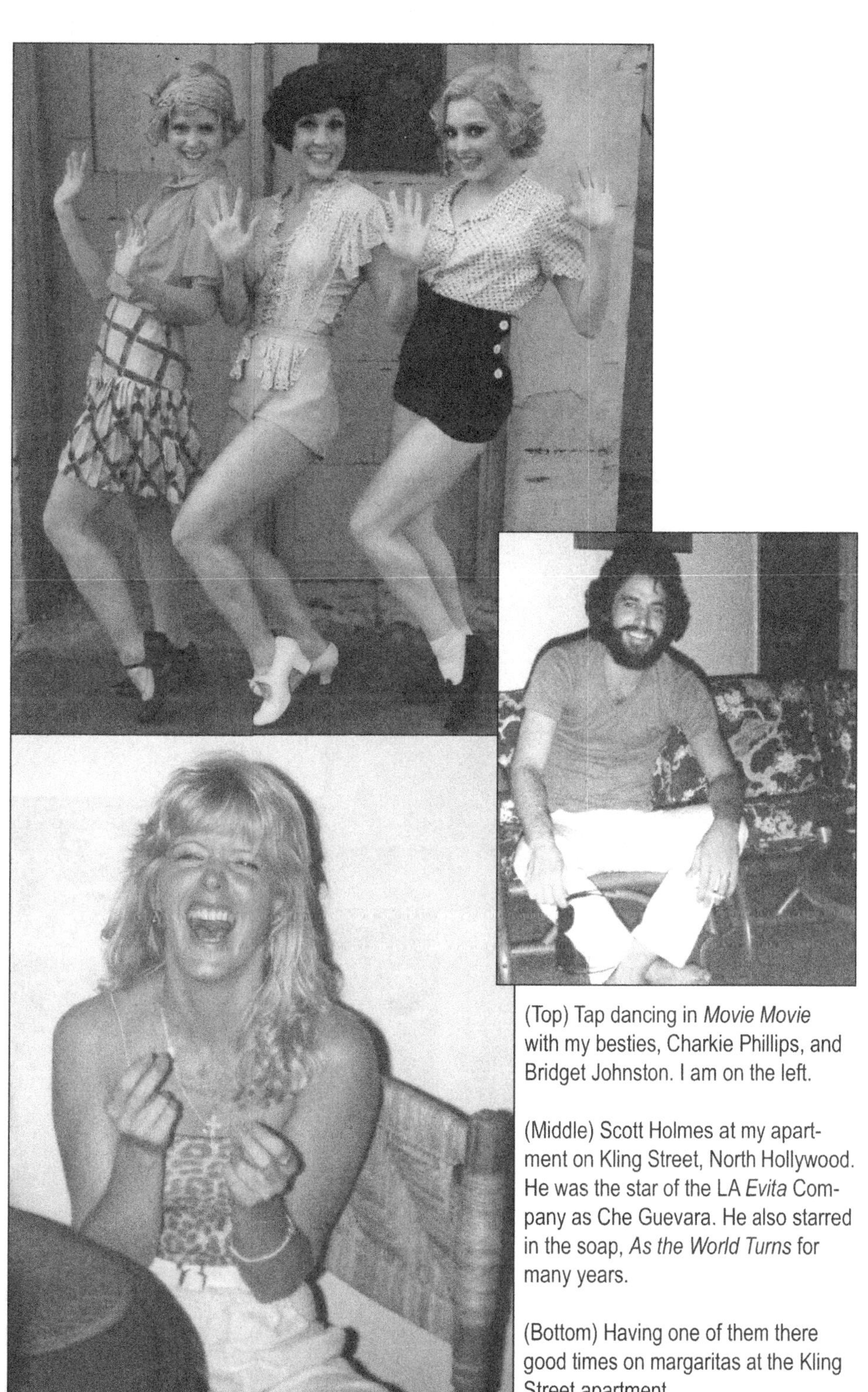

(Top) Tap dancing in *Movie Movie* with my besties, Charkie Phillips, and Bridget Johnston. I am on the left.

(Middle) Scott Holmes at my apartment on Kling Street, North Hollywood. He was the star of the LA *Evita* Company as Che Guevara. He also starred in the soap, *As the World Turns* for many years.

(Bottom) Having one of them there good times on margaritas at the Kling Street apartment.

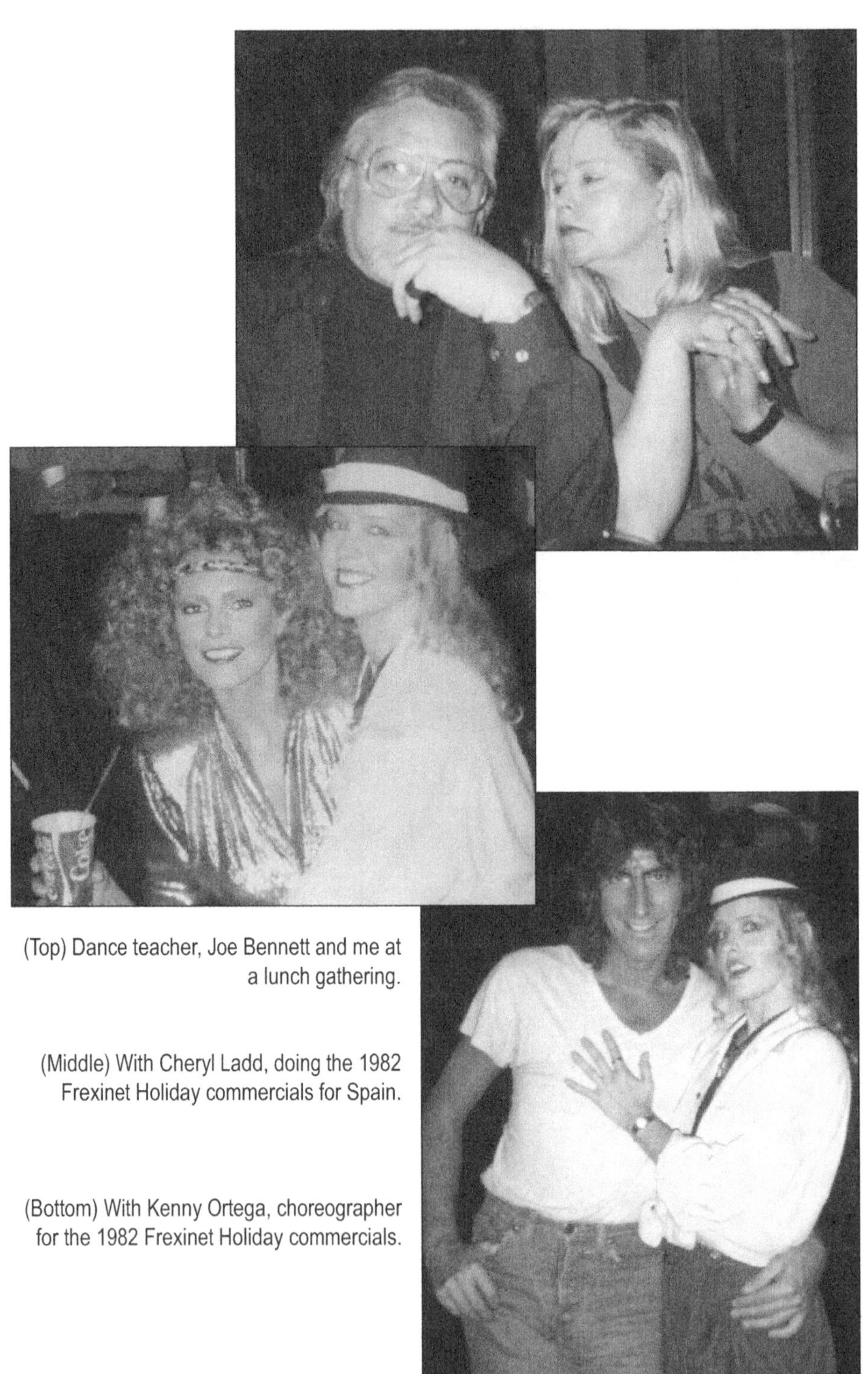

(Top) Dance teacher, Joe Bennett and me at a lunch gathering.

(Middle) With Cheryl Ladd, doing the 1982 Frexinet Holiday commercials for Spain.

(Bottom) With Kenny Ortega, choreographer for the 1982 Frexinet Holiday commercials.

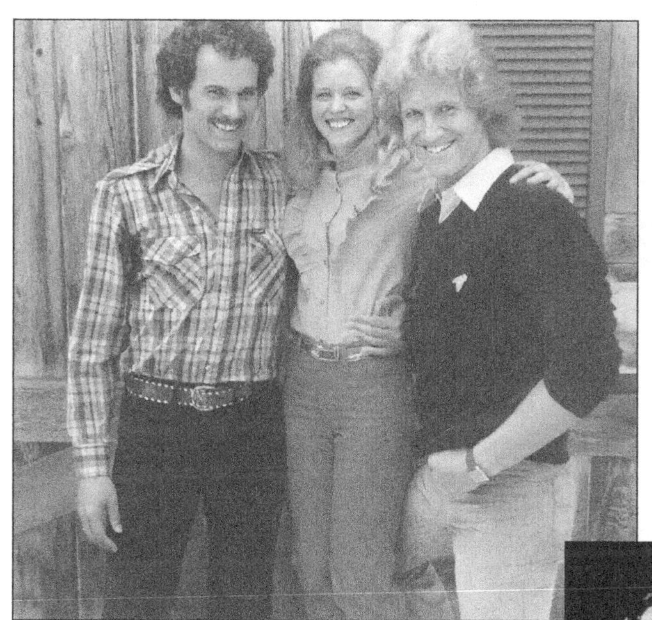

(Top) Wrangler jeans national commercial with D.J. Carroll and my partner, Michael Ragan 1982

(Middle) Pete Menefee, costumer extraordinaire, for the Debby Boone Special, One Step Closer, and yours truly. 1982

(Bottom) Me in "Dance, Dance, Dance", Debby Boone Special 1982

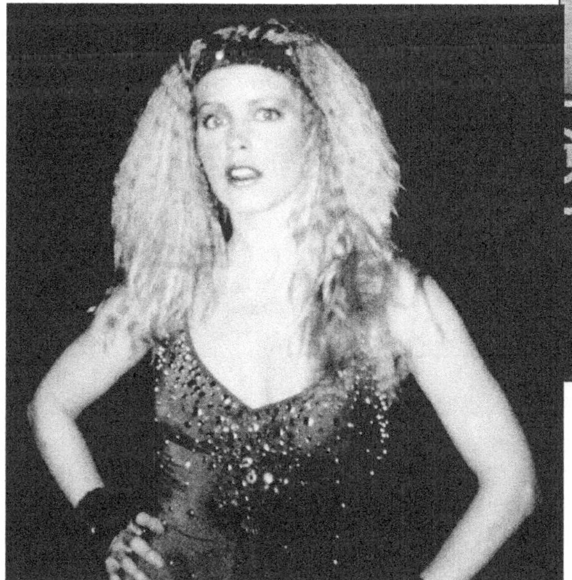

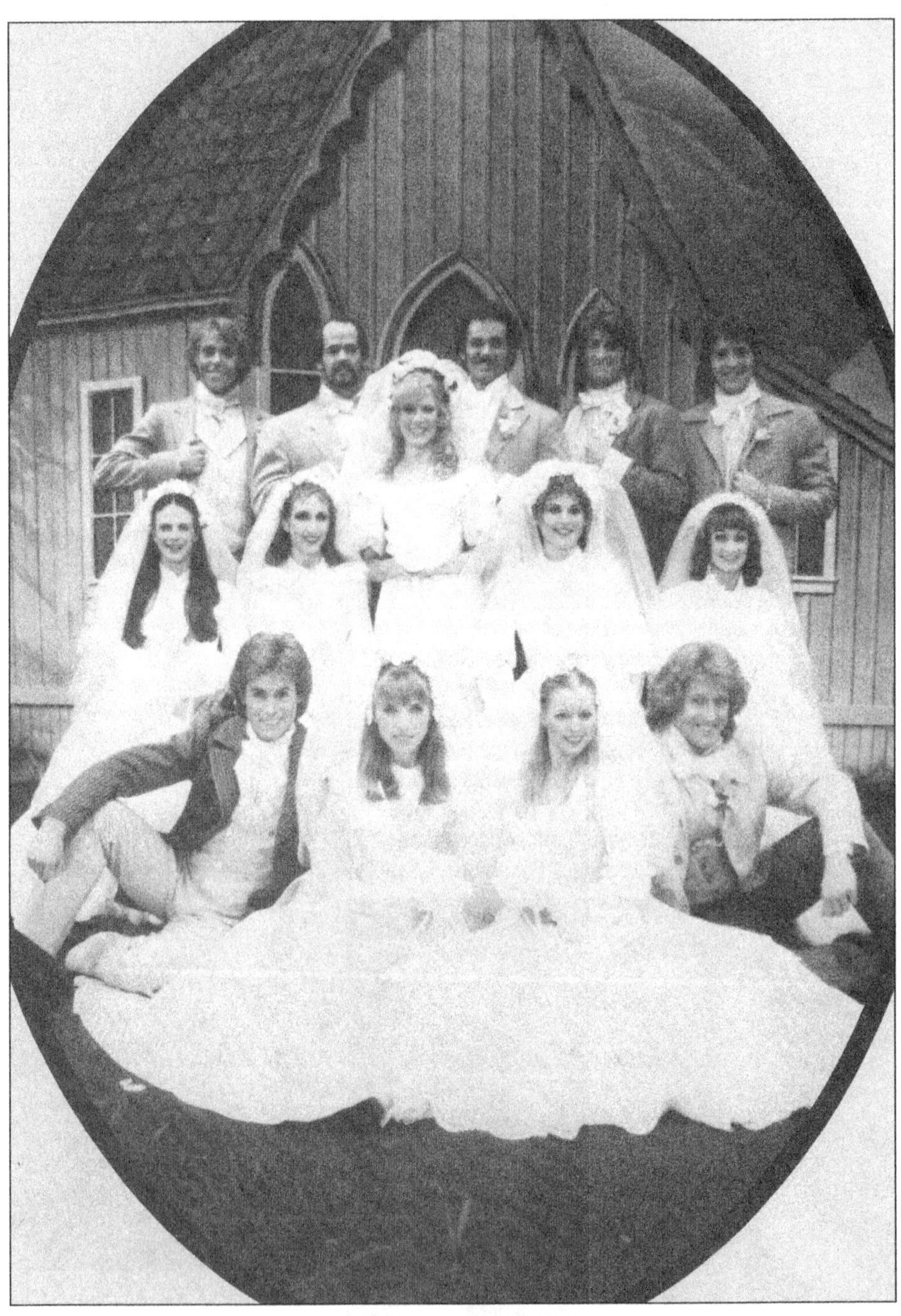

Top of photo *Seven Brides for Seven Brothers* Original Broadway cast.1982
Bottom of photo: Top left to right, Lara Teeter, D. Scott Davidge, D. J. Carrol, Jeff Calhoun, Jeffrey Reynolds, Middle, left to right, Sha Newman, Manette LaChance, Debby Boone, Jani Mussetter, Laurel van der Linde, Bottom, left to right, Craig Peralta, Nancy Fox, me, and dance partner, Michael Ragan.

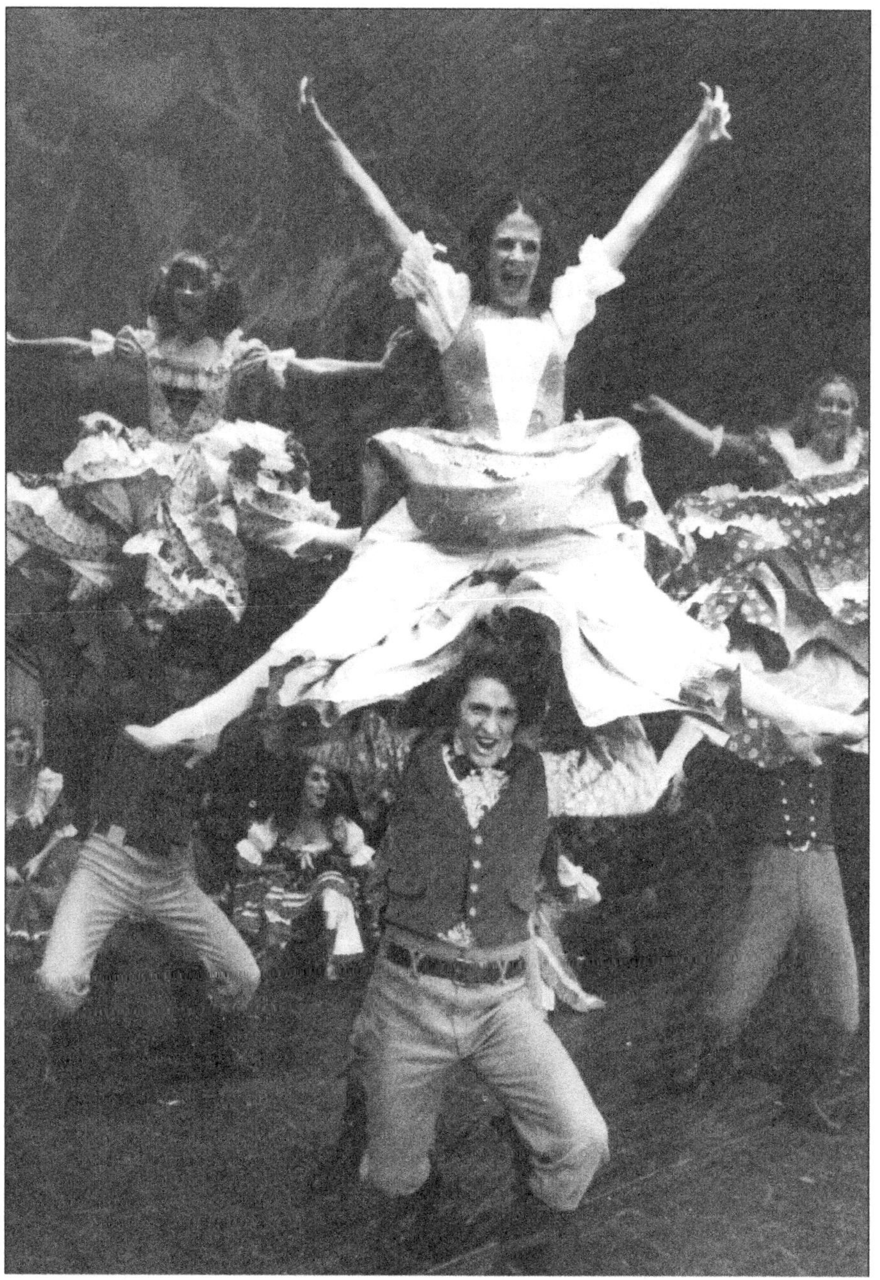

The toss and snatch lift. *Seven Brides for Seven Brothers*. In the air left to right, Laurel van der Linde, Sha Newman, me. Under Sha, front, Jeffrey Reynolds.

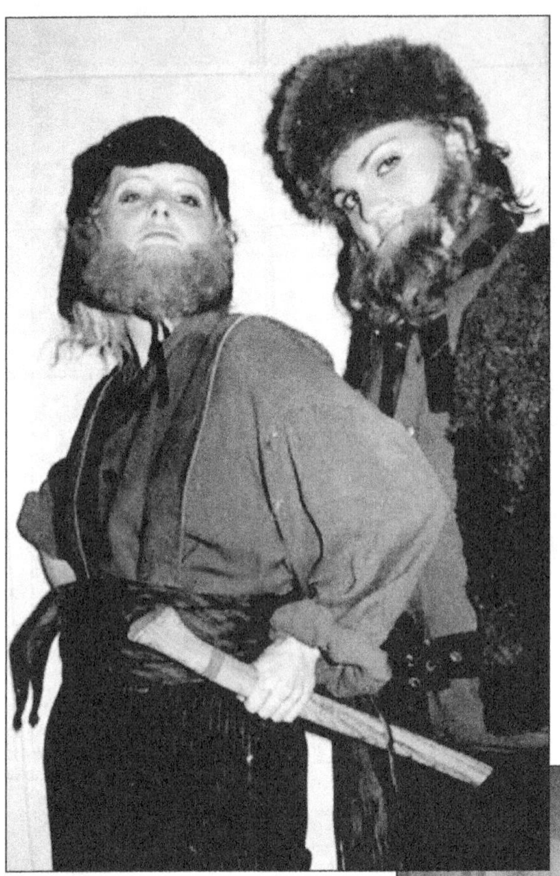

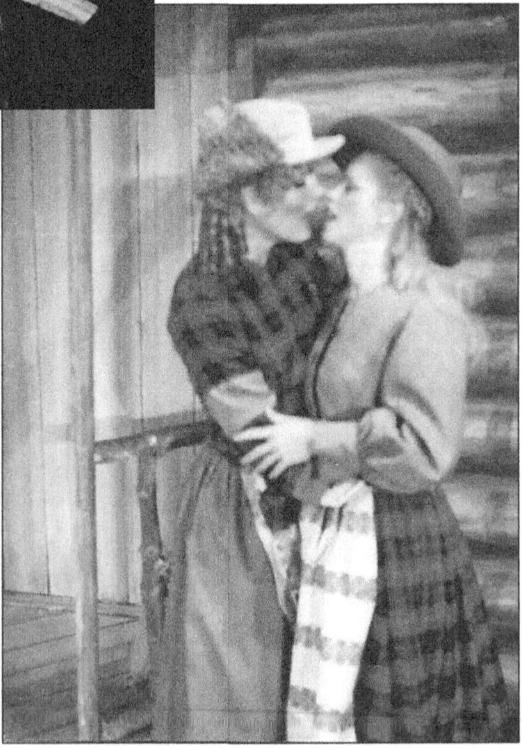

(Top) Jani Mussetter and me backstage *Seven Brides for Seven Brothers*, as lumberjacks, hijinks and tomfoolery.

(Right) Jani Mussetter and me in the winter scene, *Seven Brides for Seven Brothers*. Brides will be girls!

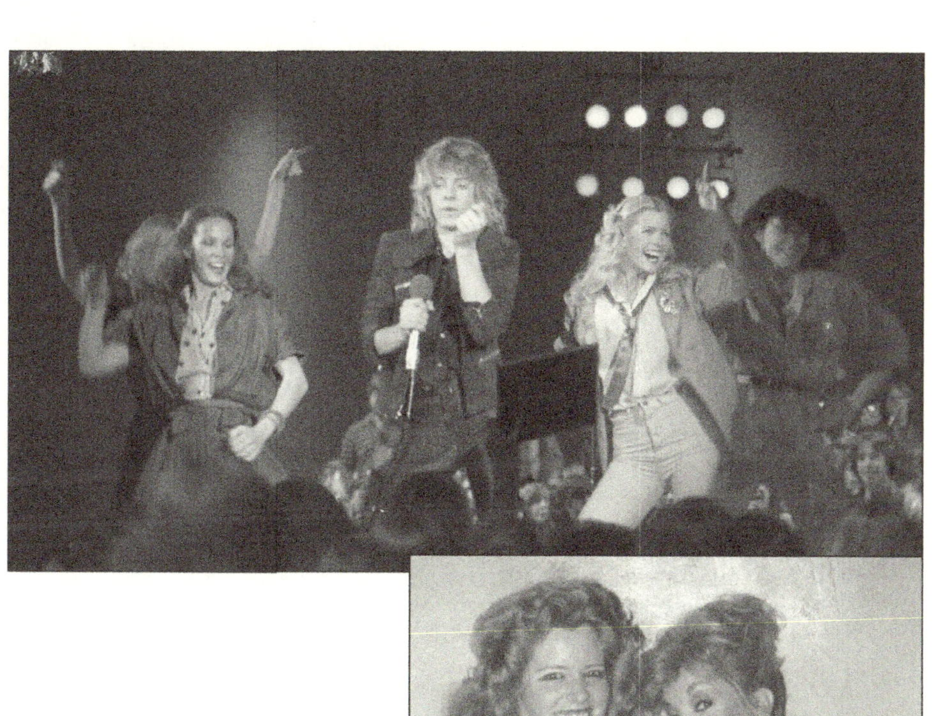

(Top) *The Leif Garrett TV Special*, dancing with Leif.
1979

(Middle) Final cast of *Seven Brides for Seven Brothers*, starring Stella Parton, at San Bernardino Civic Light Opera.
1983

(Bottom) My last Frankincense, Blaine Savage, San Bernardino Civic Light Opera.
1983

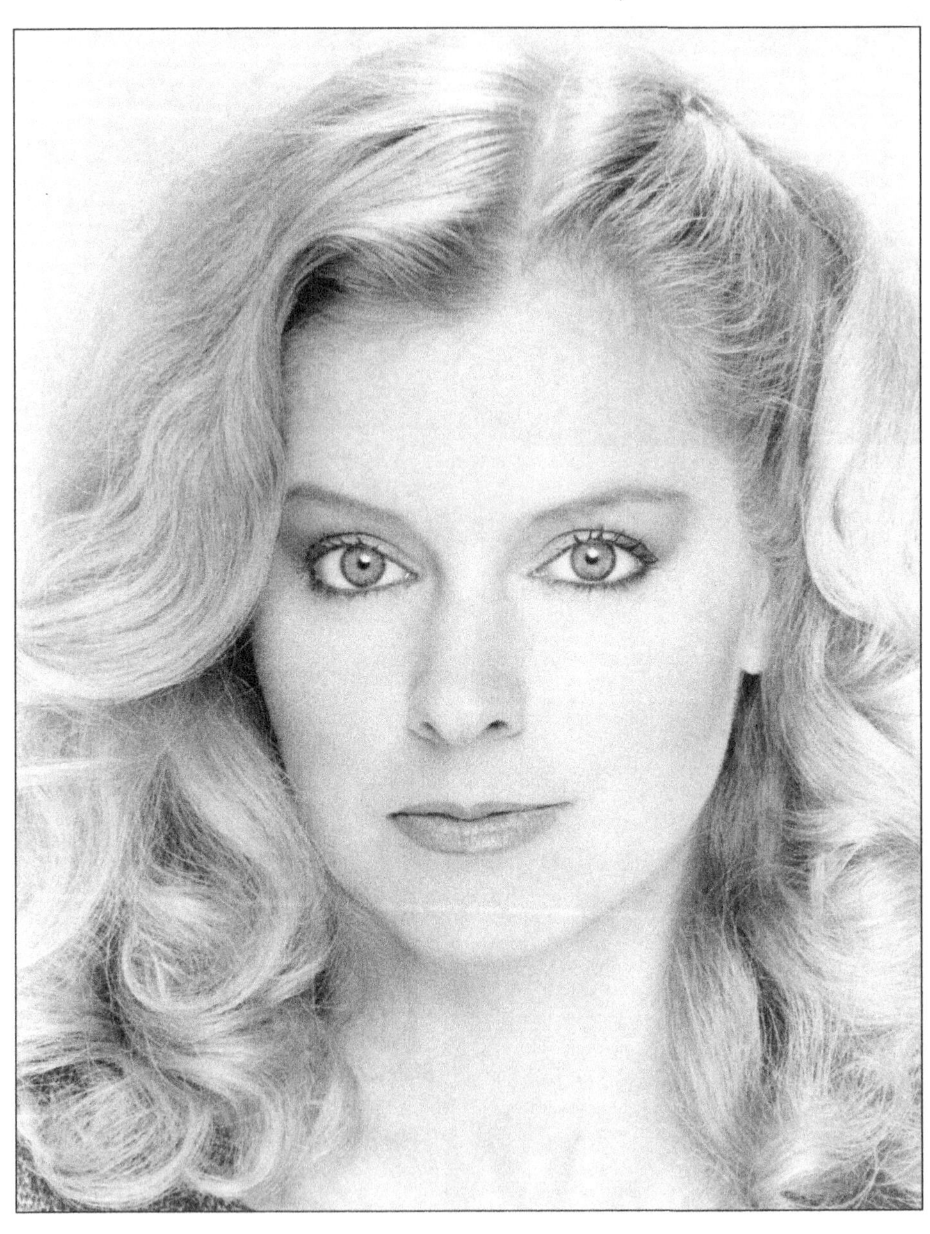

New York City Headshot by Marc Raboy.
1982

REFERENCES

Love to Love You Brady's, The Bizarre Story of The Brady Bunch Variety Hour
Authors: Susan Olson, Ted Nichelson, and Lisa Sutton
2009 published by ECW Press

Don't Panic
Author: Debra Keener
2019 published by Create Space Independent Publishing Platform

Secrets of Playboy
Documentary 2022
Director: Alexandra Dean, featuring Sondra Theodore
Streaming on Prime Video

Made in the USA
Coppell, TX
15 November 2025